MEASURING HEALTH AND MEDICAL OUTCOMES

MEASURING HEALTH AND MEDICAL OUTCOMES

Series editor
Martin Bulmer

Additional titles to include:

Measuring health and medical outcomes

Edited by

Crispin Jenkinson
University of Oxford

First published in 1994 by UCL Press
UCL Press Limited
University College London
Gower Street
London WC1E 6BT

The name of University College London (UCL) is a registered
trade mark used by UCL Press with the consent of the owner.

ISBN:
1-85728-083-0 HB
1-85728-084-9 PB

British Library Cataloguing-in-Publication Data
A CIP catalogue record for this book is available from the British Library.

Library of Congress Cataloging-in-Publication Data
Measuring health and medical outcomes/edited by Crispin Jenkinson.
   p.   cm. — (Social research today series: v.3)
   Includes bibliographical references and index.
   ISBN 1-85728-083-0 : $75.00. — ISBN 1-85728-084-9 (pbk.) : $29.95
   1. Health surveys.   I. Jenkinson, Crispin, 1962–   II. Series
RA408.5.M44   1994
610′.723–dc20   94-12568
                                                                              CIP .

Typeset in Palatino.
Printed and bound by
Biddles Ltd, Guildford and King's Lynn, England.

Contents

CONTENTS

Acknowledgements

A number of people have contributed to this book either directly or indirectly, and I owe a very real debt of thanks to Ray Fitzpatrick, Sue Ziebland, Angela Coulter and Caroline Fennell for their help and support over the past year and a half.

I am fortunate in having worked within the Health Services Research Unit in Oxford, where an enormous amount of support and help has been forthcoming. I would particularly like to thank Lucie Wright, Viv Peto, Diana Harwood and Peter Brooks for their intellectual support as well as help in preparing the text for publication. The Health Services Research Unit is part of the University Department of Public Health and Primary Care, and within that department I wish to thank Professor Martin Vessey for help and support. I am also indebted to J. A. Muir Gray, Director of Health Policy and Public Health at Oxford Regional Health Authority, for his encouragement for this venture. Within the academic community at large I would like to thank John Brazier, Nick Black, Muriel Egerton, Michael Argyle, Hannah McGee, John Ware and David Radosevich for their time and expertise at various points during the production of this text.

I wish to thank various institutions and their representatives for material help and permission to produce copyrighted questionnaires in this text. I am grateful to Nuffield College for financial support during the early stages of this project, and to John Ware, trustee of the Medical Outcomes Trust, for permitting me to reproduce the SF-36, Anne Damiano of John Hopkins University for permission to reproduce the Sickness Impact Profile (reproduced here as the Anglicized version, the Functional Limitations Profile) and Deborah Johnson of The Dartmouth COOP Project, for permitting me to reproduce the Dartmouth COOP Charts.

I also owe a real debt of thanks to Paul Montgomery, Charles Duncan and Ralph Dennison for their unfailing support. Finally, I wish to thank my parents, to whom I owe, of course, the greatest debt: this book is dedicated to them.

Contributors

Gary Albrecht PhD, Professor, School of Public Health, University of Illinois, Chicago.

Martin Bardsley PhD, Health Intelligence Manager, North Thames Regional Health Authority.

Matthew G. Clayton BA, Lecturer, Department of Government, Brunel University.

Ray Fitzpatrick PhD, Fellow, Nuffield College, Oxford, and University Lecturer in Medical Sociology, Department of Public Health and Primary Care, University of Oxford.

Andrew M. Garratt MSc, Research Assistant, Health Services Research Unit, Department of Public Health, University of Aberdeen.

Crispin Jenkinson DPhil, Deputy Director, Health Services Research Unit, Department of Public Health and Primary Care, University of Oxford.

Kate Lawrence MB BS MSc, MRC Research Fellow, Health Services Research Unit, Department of Public Health and Primary Care, University of Oxford.

Kathy Rowan DPhil, Director, Intensive Care National Audit and Research Centre, London.

Danny A. Ruta MFPHM, Consultant in Public Health Medicine, Tayside Health Board, Dundee.

Andrew D. Williams BA, Lecturer, Department of Philosophy, University of York.

Simon J. Williams PhD, Lecturer, Department of Sociology, University of Warwick.

Lucie Wright MSc, Research Fellow, Academic Department of Psychiatry, Royal Free Hospital School of Medicine, University of London.

Sue Ziebland MSc, Senior Research Fellow, ICRF General Practice Research Group, Department of Public Health and Primary Care, University of Oxford.

CHAPTER 1
Measuring health and medical outcomes: an overview

Crispin Jenkinson

Health, illness and disease

Medical intervention is intended, for the most part, to maintain or improve functioning and wellbeing, and subsequently to improve quality of life. While such a view may seem unremarkable the medical profession has not traditionally undertaken systematic evaluation of the impact of medical care from the patients' perspective. Undeniably, doctors have often asked patients if they were feeling better or worse, but the attempt to build this into a standardized metric that could take its place beside laboratory and radiological data, or beside morbidity and mortality statistics, is a relatively recent phenomenon. Traditionally a dichotomy has existed between a biomedical model and a more holistic view of health, which includes aspects of emotional and social wellbeing and functioning.

The biomedical model of ill health is rooted in a belief that ill health is an objective, measurable state. This is a disease-based view of ill health, in which poor health is a function of an abnormality. As Field (1976) remarks, the term disease is invariably used in a limited and scientific sense. Illness, on the other hand, refers to a person's subjective experience of "ill health" and is indicated by reported symptoms and subjective accounts in terms of pain, distress, discomfort, and the like. Increasingly, however, there has grown a disillusionment with the purely biomedical model of health assessment, and interest has grown in attempting to supplement such data with subjective patient-based evaluations.

The attempt to evaluate health, and the impact of medical interventions on health, purely in terms of the traditional "objective disease-based" model has become unpopular for broadly three reasons (Macintyre

1

1986a). First, the attempt to develop objective standards of assessment, with cut-off points indicating abnormality, has met with only limited success. For example, blood tests may indicate elevated erythrocyte sedimentation rate, low haemoglobin count and raised platelet count. Such results may suggest the presence of illness, most likely in the form of rheumatoid arthritis, but this may not be supported by clinical judgement. Similarly, blood pressure may be viewed as "high" for a given individual who never develops any other signs of "ill health". Related to this issue, is the second difficulty in adopting an "objective disease-based" model, namely the frequently reported discord between subjective accounts of health, and traditional medical measures. There is wide variation in reported feelings of ill health, and this bears only some relation to underlying disease state. It is, for example, possible to feel ill without any signs of underlying disease, and possible to have disease without any subjective awareness of illness. General practitioners are only too well aware of the numerous arrivals at their doors, who complain of dizziness, fatigue, nausea, pain, weakness, etc., yet for whom no underlying organic symptoms can be detected. Similarly, many people with serious illnesses either ignore the symptoms, regard them as part of day-to-day life, or are completely unaware of any problems. At the extreme end of this spectrum, Melzack (1973) documents the case of a patient who, despite extensive skin and bone trauma, was, for the most part, unaware of her condition. Only during the last month of her life did this patient report feeling discomfort and pain. Similarly, Williams, in a study of patients with chronic respiratory illness, found that spirometric measures of lung function were only weakly related to breathlessness, physical disability and psychosocial aspects of quality of life (Williams 1993). Thus, "objectively" defined disease does not bear a simple causal relationship with subjectively experienced illness. Thirdly, it has been suggested that certain forms of objectively defined diseases may be so prevalent that they are rarely viewed as illnesses by those who experience them. For example, Norton et al. (1988) in a study of women with incontinence, found a considerable delay in their seeking medical help, and that 11 per cent of the respondents had thought the problem were "normal". Thus, while surveys of the general populations have tended to indicate that most respondents view their health as good, and do not report any ailments, illnesses are present in quite substantial numbers, and hence never reach the doctor's door. As Macintyre notes, "Screening studies of random cross sections of the population have tended to show that very few people are without some abnormalities that can be defined as disease, even though many of the affected individuals are unaware of the disorders." By way of example Macintyre cites the Peckham Experiment in the 1930s, in which health overhauls were conducted on 1,206 families (4,002 individuals). The results indicated that discoverable pathological conditions were present in the majority (approximately 90%) of the sample, yet for those in whom disorders were detected, only around 30% were aware of them (Pearse & Crocker 1943, Macintyre 1986b). Furthermore, evidence suggests that while individuals may experience long term illnesses or disabilities, and be aware of them, results indicate such people also report their health as good. Such have been the findings in the UK General Household Survey, conducted every year since 1971, and in many surveys on health and lifestyles undertaken in recent years. For example, in the Oxford Healthy Lifestyles Survey (Wright et al. 1992) only 12% of respondents claimed their health was "fair" or "poor" in response to the question "In general, would you say your health is Excellent, Very Good, Good, Fair or Poor?". However, the same survey revealed 30% of the respondents, from their own self report, to have chronic illnesses or longstanding disabilities. Indeed, of those reporting long term chronic illness only 28% reported their health as fair or poor. This survey strikingly highlights the complexities of assessing health. On the one hand, individuals may actually be fully aware of their disease state, and yet, on the other hand, see their overall health as good. Such an apparently counter-intuitive finding highlights the difficulty of measuring health status. In part, such results indicate the myriad of meanings that people attach to the term "health".

Herzlich (1973), from a pioneering study on lay concepts of health and disease, found that health was regarded as multidimensional: the absence of disease, a positive state of wellbeing, and a "reserve" of overall health, determined in large part by individual constitution. Subsequent studies have tended to broadly support these findings (Pill & Stott 1982, Blaxter 1985). However, despite the tendency to characterize health in a largely positive manner, individuals also have the ability to define health as co-existing with serious and/or long term illnesses (Blaxter 1990). For those intent on measuring health, then, there is no simple solution: individuals are perfectly capable of admitting to serious long term illness and yet claiming to be healthy; to report symptoms and yet have no discoverable pathology, and to be assessed by the medical profession as diseased, and yet experience no negative symptoms. It is an increasing awareness of the limitations of traditional measures of health, and an increasing belief that individuals have important knowledge of their own health state (Tuckett et al. 1985), which should be carefully monitored and recorded, that has fuelled the search for subjective health measures. In the final analysis, treatments that lead to successful removal of disease and yet do not improve quality of life or health status can be viewed as having succeeded in only a rather limited technical and medical sense.

The scope of this book

This volume attempts to address the complex methodological and theoretical issues that surround the measurement of health from the perspective of the patient. The purpose of the text is twofold. On the one hand it is intended that it should act as an introduction to the field, and provide an outline to the potential uses and benefits of subjective accounts of health. On the other hand, it is intended to provide a critical commentary on potential difficulties in the use of such data.

Epidemiologists, clinicians and medical researchers are now only too well aware that quality of life must in some way be measured. With increasing concern as to the efficacy of treatments, patients, to a much greater extent, are being asked to report their own health status, in a way that can be analyzed quantitatively, and in such a way that will inform medical practice. In a relatively short period of time, questionnaires designed to assess subjective health status measures have become a valued aspect of medical evaluation and their potential benefits advocated.

The history of the development of health status measurement is documented in this book by Gary Albrecht, while the potential uses of such data are outlined by Ray Fitzpatrick. The remaining chapters discuss methodological issues that have tended to be overlooked or dealt with only briefly in most texts dealing with health status measurement.

An increasing use of measures of health status is in evaluating change over time. In her chapter, Sue Ziebland discusses potential ways in which existing measures may provide very different pictures of change, and suggests that the reason for this is in large part due to the differing models of disability underlying the construction of the various measures. The chapter highlights the need for caution when selecting measures, and advice on how appropriate measures are selected and longitudinal designs conducted. One major concern of those considering using such measures is the time taken to complete many health status measures. Kathy Rowan provides a review of the potential uses and limitations of global measures and short-form instruments. The amount of measurement precision that may be lost with global measures or domains in questionnaires constructed from single items, is discussed, and the potential uses of such data, for example in routine evaluation, is outlined. Evidence suggests that data from such simple measures can be both informative and reliable. The chapters by Crispin Jenkinson, Lucie Wright, and Simon Williams, address psychometric issues relating to the three most frequently used generic health status measures. Crispin Jenkinson outlines the way in which questionnaires are designed and items weighted for severity. He then discusses how the most complex of these methods was utilised to develop item weights for the Nottingham Health Profile. Although this questionnaire has undergone considerable psychometric testing and validation the scheme used to weight items can cause inaccuracies, and the format of the questionnaire can be difficult for respondents to complete. In part it is for these reasons that interest has shifted to the "short-form" measures originating from research originally undertaken by the RAND Corporation of America. Lucie Wright documents the development of the short-form measures, and outlines the various ways in which the original SF-20, a 20-item health status instrument, was validated, and then replaced, due to psychometric limitations, with the SF-36, containing 36 items. Simon Williams provides a detailed history of the development and validation of the Sickness Impact Profile, and its UK counterpart, the Functional Limitations Profile. These measures tend to be viewed as "gold standards", by which other measures may be assessed, but they do have limitations.

Danny Ruta and Andrew Garratt adopt an entirely different approach to the measurement of health status, arguing that the primary purpose of medical care is to improve quality of life, and this should be measured directly. They suggest a new approach to the measurement of health status, whereby each individual is asked to nominate areas of life which have been adversely affected by ill health, and then to indicate the extent of the impact. The results from this procedure provide an index figure of "quality of life". At odds with the views of Ruta and Garratt, Matthew Clayton and Andrew Williams argue that the purpose of medical care is not primarily to improve welfare or quality of life, but capabilities. The possible implications of attempts to measure "welfare" are discussed.

The final chapter provides an overview of the text, intending to bring together the various themes of the book, and outlining potential future issues on the research agenda. A glossary of frequently used terms in the area are to be found in an appendix.

CHAPTER 2

Subjective health assessment

Gary L. Albrecht

Introduction

One of the anomalies in contemporary medical practice is that patients' perceptions of personal health, wellbeing and life satisfaction are often discordant with their objective health status. Some individuals in seemingly good health report that they do not feel well, are lonely, and cannot go out in the community or work (Blazer & Houpt 1979, Gallagher in press, Imershein et al. in press). Others with serious medical problems and activity limitations rank their health equal to or better than their peers and say that they are satisfied with the quality of their lives (Stoller 1984, Goldstein & Hurwicz 1989). Clearly, then, health involves something more than is captured in objective measures of morbidity, mortality and activity limitations. For these reasons, subjective health assessment is a critically important component of contemporary health services research and clinical practice.

This chapter situates the subjective assessment of health in current medical practice and health services research. The chapter emphasizes the importance of understanding and measuring patients' perceptions of their health in determining health status. Next, the chapter traces the historical development of subjective health assessment in health services research. Then, the chapter examines the content domains of questionnaires and instruments designed to measure perceptions of health status and discusses the validity of using subjective health experiences to assess health status. Finally, techniques are suggested for closing the gaps between theory and practice in using subjective indicators to assess health status and apply the results to clinical practice and policy initiatives.

The importance of subjective health assessment

The practice of Western medicine is germ theory oriented and tech-
nologically driven. As a consequence, physicians employ sophisticated
scientific equipment and procedures to search for the organic bases of
disease in making their differential diagnoses (Gelijns & Thier 1990).
Likewise, in formulating treatment plans, physicians are taught to rely
on the most recent technology in attacking pathology with effective
interventions that can meet a scientific standard; that is, that either have
been or can be demonstrated to be efficacious in clinical trials (Gelijns
1990). Physicians are further instructed to supplement their use of tests
with a social history taken from patients and/or their family and
friends. Taken together, the test results, socio-demographic data and self
reports constitute a set of objective and subjective indicators called
symptoms and signs that are used to construct the total diagnostic picture (Muller 1990, Wilson et al. 1991).

The bias of scientific medicine is to prefer objective test results over
subjective personal reports in determining an accurate diagnosis (Albert
et al. 1988). With clinical experience, however, physicians often realize
that social histories and personal reports are invaluable sources of data
in ascertaining the epidemiology of a condition, the nature of the com-
plaint, available resources and the types of treatment most preferred by
the patient (Waitzkin 1991). In addition, evidence shows that patients
often do not comply with prescribed treatments unless they are actively
included in the therapeutic process, understand their condition and
therapy, have the resources to carry out the course of treatment and are
motivated to do so (Stanton 1987, Villar et al. 1991). For these reasons, an
objective and subjective understanding of illness is imperative in the
diagnosis and treatment of illness and disability (Herzlich & Pierret
1987). Until recently, more attention was given to the objective determination of pathology and illness than to subjective health assessment.
However, this imbalance is rapidly changing.

Ironically, recent emphasis on health care reform in the United States
and Britain, embodying different forms of managed competition and a
revolution in health services research focusing on medical outcomes,
have serendipitously turned attention to consumer preferences and subjective health assessment (Starr 1992). Until health care costs became
unbearable in the United States and a growing burden in Britain, gov-
ernments and providers delivered goods and services according to what

medical experts deemed necessary or wealthy consumers would purchase. Government and health care providers generally assumed that if the infrastructures were adequate, delivery processes monitored and sufficient resources allocated, the nation's health problems would be under control. Under this model, government officials and medical experts decided what was good for the nation's health. Science, objectivity and technology dominated their values and perspective. In the traditional systems, consumers did not have power even approximating that of other major stakeholders in health care transactions.

This traditional system of health care delivery is undergoing substantial re-assessment and change. Rapidly rising costs of care without corresponding decreases in disability, morbidity and mortality turned expert attention to cost–benefit analyses of health care (Ellwood 1988, Enthoven 1993). Government, employers and consumers want demonstrated value for the money they spend on health care. Influenced by these trends, Wennberg and his associates strongly supported a US Congressional initiative to mandate that the Agency for Health Care Policy and Research promote research on medical outcomes and develop guidelines for practice (Wennberg 1990a). Medical outcomes research arose when Wennberg noticed considerable regional and practice differences in rates for surgical procedures such as prostatectomy and coronary bypasses even when controlling for severity of the condition, patient health and socio-demographic characteristics (Wennberg 1990b). Sometimes these rates varied by factors of 5 to 8 times more in one geographic region or practice than in another and for no apparent reason. To investigate these puzzling disparities, Wennberg and associates began focusing on what works in medicine and on learning how "to make clinical decisions that reflect more truly the needs and wants of individual patients" (Wennberg 1990a). Patients were involved as key actors in outcomes research because they were recognized as critical contributors to their own diagnosis and treatment. In pilot programmes on outcomes research, patients were asked to provide information about symptoms, functional status, health perceptions and feelings concerning their health, perceived problems and proposed treatment alternatives. After these interviews and medical work-ups, the patient was given a diagnosis, proposed treatment alternatives and estimated probabilities of likely outcome. The patient was then actively assisted in making a decision on therapy. In these pilot efforts, subjective health assessment was a fundamental component in formulating diagnoses and treatment plans.

This approach is based on the assumptions that patients often know what is wrong, what is best for their recovery and what treatment regimens they are likely to follow with commitment. These assumptions are supported by preliminary evidence. Research shows that patients often assess their diagnosis and measure their "successes" against personal life course and disease trajectories, previous personal experience and the experience of their peers (Markson et al. 1991, Albrecht & Levy 1991, Anspach 1991). Also, patients often are good judges of how they will do in therapy and what suits them best (Albrecht 1976, Albrecht & Higgins 1977).

Indeed, an accumulating body of cross-cultural evidence indicates that patients and aging people are insightful judges of their own health, morbidity and mortality. In a number of studies in the United States, Japan and Scandinavian countries ageing persons with serious health conditions were frequently better judges of their future functional status and likelihood of mortality than were experts (Haga et al. 1993, Dean 1993, Marshall 1993). When individuals were asked to assess their general level of health, they were able to do so without difficulty. Furthermore, experts were startled to learn that these self assessments of health were often powerful predictors of mortality even when they were controlled for many other clinical, life course and socio-demographic variables (Birren 1993). Similar efforts in institutional research demonstrate that patients are also informative and useful evaluators of the care they receive in the hospital (Cleary et al. 1991). Both the health outcomes movement and studies on the power of health perceptions to explain morbidity and mortality events and hospital care outcomes underline the importance of carefully considering subjective health assessment in health services research, clinical practice and social policy. An historical review demonstrates how the field grew, what was accomplished, and the problems that were addressed.

Historical development of subjective health assessment

Interest in subjective health assessment is a relatively recent phenomenon which developed concurrently with research on quality of life and subjective wellbeing. Subjective health assessment asks people to report on their own health, illnesses and functional status. Such assessments can focus on physical or mental health or a combination of both. Subjective wellbeing and subjective health assessment historically are subsumed under the broader quality of life concept which includes measures of health, function, resources, happiness, life satisfaction and positive affect; many of which are measured in terms of subjective perceptions (Diener 1984). Searches of social science and medical reference data bases indicate that literature on subjective health assessment is most often found under the key words "health quality of life". In fact, there are few references to subjective health assessment in large data bases like Social Science Abstracts and Medline. The evolution of the subjective health assessment techniques, then, takes place within the historical context of quality of life research.

The first known reference to quality of life is in A. C. Pigou's *The Economics of Welfare* (1920) where he discusses government support for the poor in terms of personal wellbeing and the national dividend. The Oxford English Dictionary (OED 1982) first notes the use of "quality of life" in J. B. Priestly's work, *Daylight on Saturday*, "The plans are already . . . maturing that would give all our citizens more security, better opportunities and a nobler quality of life" (1943). In a similar vein, Arthur Schlesinger observed in the *New York Times Magazine*, "The liberal's belief in working for change does . . . mean that he feels history can never stand still, that social change can better the quality of people's lives and happiness, and that the margin of change, however limited, is worth the effort" (4 March 1956: 60/3). In these usages, the OED says that "quality" refers to the capability, ability or skill of a person or to an attribute, property or special feature of a thing. Quality of life in early academic literature and the press, then, referred to the capability and wellbeing of an individual and by extension to a general population.

Academic interest in quality of life was stimulated by the social inequalities in Western societies which, when publicly acknowledged after the Second World War, gave impetus to the social movements of the 1960s. Recognition of social inequities and the evolution of the welfare state in Scandinavia and subsequently in Europe and the United States sparked a literature on social indicators and subjective wellbeing in the 1970s. Drewnowski (1974) and Erickson (1974) both pioneered quality of life and welfare state analyses in Europe. Researchers at the University of Michigan (Andrews & Withey 1976, Campbell et al. 1976) spearheaded studies examining quality of work, family and leisure life in the American context.

A computerized search of Medline reveals that health-related quality of life was first mentioned in the medical literature in 1966 by J. R. Elkinton in an article of the *Annals of Internal Medicine*, "Medicine and the Quality of Life". The results of the entire search are summarized in Table 2.1.

Table 2.1 Number of references to health related quality of life in MEDLINE, 1966–1993.

Years	Number of references
1966–1974	40
1975–1980	1,309
1981–1985	1,907
1986–1990	5,078
1991–May 1993	4936

The exponential growth in literature on health related quality of life over the last 33 years is striking. A review of randomly selected articles reveals that subjective health assessment is a major component of these papers which generally concentrate on treatment effectiveness as measured by the prolongation of life, alleviation of distress and restoration of function and wellbeing (Tarlov 1983, Ellwood 1988). These papers reflect the growing interest of physicians and health researchers in utilizing the patient's viewpoint in formulating treatment plans and monitoring the quality of medical care outcomes (Geigle & Jones 1990). As Ware (1992) observes: "Although the patient is the best source of information regarding the achievement of these goals, information from patients about their experiences of disease and treatment has not been routinely collected in clinical research or medical practice." He and many others obviously believe that it is important to include subjective health assessments as integral parts of research and clinical practice and are doing so. Experts and the lay public alike, then, became increasingly concerned with health related quality of life as more of the population experienced the inexorable limitations of ageing, chronic illness and disability, realized the consequences of prolonging life in a diminished condition through technological interventions, searched for a more humanistic form of health care and grappled with the escalating costs of medical care (Levine 1987, Johnson & Wolinsky 1993).

Interest in health-related quality of life and by implication subjective health assessment also is congruent with the World Health Organisation's definition of health: "Health is a state of complete physical, mental and social wellbeing and not merely the absence of disease or infirmity" (WHO 1947). This definition underscores the importance of including the functional, social, cultural, subjective and social-psychological variables that impact on rôle performance, independent living and perceived wellbeing in any elaborated conception of health (Bury 1982, Katz 1987). Later a WHO scientific group added that personal "autonomy" was also critical to quality of life (WHO 1984).

Health-related quality of life is a concept that attempts to encompass the spirit of the WHO definition of health by incorporating both personal health status and social wellbeing in assessing the health of individuals and populations (Guyatt et al. 1993). The concept has not been well defined because it evolved from a loosely integrated body of research on health status, functional performance and social wellbeing. This body of work assimilated studies of physical conditions like diagnostic category, health status, and functional ability; psychological factors like pain, emotions, locus of control, sense of self worth and intellectual functioning; social variables like social rôle performance and support networks; and composite measures of these elements in ascertaining health-related quality of life (Bowling 1991, Larson 1993). The interrelationships of these concepts and variables are complex for social-psychological factors like self efficacy influence health status and vice versa (Grembowski 1993).

Though experts disagree on a single definition of health-related quality of life, they generally concur on the components that ought to be included (Pope & Tarlov 1991). Patrick and Erickson provide a recent example of such a definition and its component parts. "Health related quality of life is the value assigned to duration of life as modified by the impairments, functional states, perceptions and social opportunities that are influenced by disease, injury, treatment, or policy" (1993). Five core dimensions of health-related quality of life are embodied in this definition: resilience, health perception, physical function, symptoms and duration of life. While other experts (Jette 1980, Bergner 1985, Ware 1986, Stewart 1993) use concepts like health status, cognitive function, mental health, emotional state, subjective wellbeing, life satisfaction and social support to characterize and assess health-related quality of life, they cover much of the same ground as Patrick and Erickson but nevertheless contribute some important distinctions and emphases (Applegate et al. 1990, Bowling 1991).

Subjective health assessment or measurement of health-related quality of life is typically achieved through a battery of instruments. Generic instruments which provide a general health profile have been developed and subjected to considerable psychometric testing for measurement properties, including validity and reliability. Supplementary instruments are designed to measure more specific content like mental confusion and self esteem. In addition, specific scales, such as the Arthritis Impact Measurement Scale (AIMS) (Meenan et al. 1984), were constituted to assess functional ability within specific disease and disability groups.

The measures most commonly used to provide a broad health profile are the Sickness Impact Profile (SIP) (Bergner et al. 1981), Nottingham Health Profile (NHP) (Hunt et al. 1980), McMaster Health Index Questionnaire (MHIQ) (Sackett et al. 1977), and the Medical Outcomes Study (MOS) battery of instruments developed by the RAND Corporation for their health insurance studies (Ware et al. 1980). The MOS instruments include the SF-20 and revised SF-36 instruments which have been tested and normed in the United States and Britain (Jenkinson et al. 1993b). Each of these instruments shares subjective health assessment as a commonly held strategy for determining health status and related aspects of health quality of life. In all of these scales, respondents are asked to provide answers to such questions as: "Do you have trouble bending, lifting or stooping because of your health?" Yes/No; "I am going out less to visit people." Yes/No; "I have unbearable pain." Yes/No; and, "I feel consistently anxious and depressed." Yes/No.

Measurement, perspective, domains, and dimensions

Subjective health assessment instruments are organized to measure domains and dimensions of health-related quality of life. Measurement of conceptual domains and dimensions is one of the critical activities of science because researchers cannot make judgements about the existence of relationships among theoretical concepts and clinicians cannot make diagnoses nor carry out informed treatment unless they have accurate measures of health and illness applicable to both individuals and populations. "In its broadest sense, measurement is the assignment of numerals to objects or events according to rules" (Stevens 1951). Therefore, to measure health or illness, the researcher or clinician must assign numbers to represent the presence or absence of properties (Kerlinger 1973). The use of numbers in the measurement of health assumes that health is a concept with domains and dimensions that can be measured according to counting rules. Counting rules provide the observer with standards and procedures of how to assign numbers to objects or events.

Body temperature, for example, is a common indicator of health and illness for if the body temperature is too low for a protracted period of time, hypothermia can result and perhaps even death. If the body temperature is too high, brain damage and death can also result. Temperatures that are below or above average but not life threatening are also good indicators of anaemia or the presence of infection. To ascertain numbers useful for research or clinical practice experts must have a clear concept to measure with definable properties like body temperature, an accurate instrument like a mercury thermometer, counting rules to determine different levels of the property measured like degrees centigrade, standardized measurement procedures like placing the thermometer under the tongue while the person is at rest, and rules of correspondence that permit the observer to observe the level of mercury in a column of a thermometer and record a body temperature on a computer screen or piece of paper. Then, the individual's temperature must be analyzed and judged in terms of concepts, theory and previous observations on that individual and the more general population to judge whether or not the individual has a temperature outside the normal range, the individual's temperature has changed, and treatment is indicated. The measurement of health properties, then, is imperative for the conduct of health services research and the practice of clinical medicine. But experts recognize that the measurement of individual health perceptions requires a different perspective and measurement techniques than those designed to measure objective health conditions.

Subjective health assessment implies a perspective in which individuals report their health and illness perceptions. This approach is based on theories of the subjective experience of illness which assume that individuals experience illness in ways that cannot be measured well through objective tests and that these feelings and perceptions influence health outcomes (Fitzpatrick et al. 1984). This perspective emphasizes the importance of psyche as an overt contributor to physiological outcomes, acknowledges that individuals experience and react to illness differently and recognizes that individuals can accurately report their perceptions. Most researchers agree that a combination of objective and subjective measures of general health status and disease specific measures are desirable to provide a complete assessment of quality of life (Spilker 1990).

Fadan & Leplége (1992) contend that subjective health assessments are essential for determining quality of life and that these data have validity because certain human states are universally considered to be aversive such as pain, physical limitations and depression while others are desirable like mobility, peace of mind, feeling loved and supported. They argue that such perceptions directly impact individuals intentions and behaviours aimed at improving quality of life.

Studies which examined the relationships between objective (symptom related) and subjective (impact related) indicators of quality of life suggest that patients considered distress associated with the effects of disease on daily life to be more disturbing than the discomfort associated with their symptoms (Quirk & Jones 1990, Janson-Bjerkle et al. 1992). When patients' perceptions were considered in conjunction with objective measures of illness, judgements of severity were closely associated with feelings of depression, panic-fear and frequency of emergency department visits. This research implies that the impact of the illness on the individual and family, including the psychological and social burdens imposed by the disease, is as important as physical symptoms in determining quality of life, prescribing treatment and estimating outcome. Guess (1992) characterizes this new awareness in clinical practice: "Increasingly, we see the need to show that our products improve the functional status and overall health of the patients, and not just improve the biochemical test results. One does not treat hypertension merely because somebody happens to have an elevated blood pressure; one treats it because of what the blood pressure implies for the patient." This sensitivity to multiple determinants of health outcomes and quality of life alerts the researcher and clinician to those factors most likely to enhance wellbeing.

Accurate assessment of subjective health status is contingent on careful identification of the domains and dimensions that constitute health and health related quality of life and their grounding in theory. The principal theories used to undergird health-related quality of life research are functional theory from sociology, positive wellbeing and general quality of life theory from social psychology, utility theory from economics and decision sciences and psychophysics and psychoimmunology from psychology (Patrick & Erickson 1993). Each perspective of health-related quality of life utilizes a set of key concepts and their interrelationships to constitute a theoretical explanation. In turn, each theory focuses attention on specific concepts, domains and dimensions that must be measured to test the theory and/or serve as a foundation for diagnosis and treatment. Concepts are constructs, such as health-related quality of life, that cannot be measured directly but which serve to organize a series of empirical interventions, actions and outcomes. Each of these concepts is usually composed of domains and dimensions because complex concepts generally have multiple components. Domains refer to conceptually distinct areas which when taken together constitute the larger construct. Health-related quality of life, for example, is composed of such domains as physical functioning, cognitive functioning, self efficacy and wellbeing. Dimensions refer to subcomponents of the domains in larger concepts. Physical functioning, for example, comprises self care and mobility dimensions. Most widely used scales employ multiple items to measure each dimension, domain and concept and respondents are often given the opportunity to gradate their answers by strongly agree, agree, disagree, strongly disagree or by never, sometimes, often, always.

Historically, subjective health assessment and health quality of life research developed inductively and was not derived formally from some elaborated theory. The original work in the area was disparate and oriented towards solving pragmatic problems like measuring the physical function of young paraplegics in spinal cord rehabilitation programmes and assessing the emotional state of patients in psychotherapy. Empirical work concentrated on functional scales designed to assess morbidity and disability, especially among older people, so that appropriate intervention programmes could be established. These instruments were subsequently employed to measure changes in function and wellbeing due to interventions in rehabilitation programmes. The Katz (Katz et al. 1963), Barthel (Mahoney & Barthel 1965), Kenney (Schoening et al. 1965) and PULSES (Granger et al. 1979) were among the first widely used scales constructed to measure activities of daily living like self care and mobility. The Minnesota Multiphasic Personality Inventory (Hathaway 1942) and the Wechsler Memory scale (Wechsler 1945) were developed to measure personality adjustment and cognitive functioning which were useful in assessing reactions to trauma, head injuries and stroke. A third set of instruments including the Beck Depression Inventory (Beck et al.

1961) and the widely used Center for Epidemiologic Studies Depression Scale (CES-D) (Radloff 1977) were constructed to measure emotional states, particularly depression. The related Quality of Well-Being Scale (Kaplan et al. 1976) is used to measure positive affect and general wellbeing. A fourth set of instruments focuses more on resources and needs. These scales measure variables such as perceived support from family and friends (Procidano & Heller 1983), social networks (Stokes 1983) and needs assessment (Rossi & Freeman 1989).

Since these general scales often were not sensitive to some of the peculiarities of specific diseases and disabilities, more focused scales were tailored to these conditions. The Stanford Arthritis Center Health Assessment Questionnaire (HAQ) (Fries et al. 1980) and Patient Functioning and Satisfaction Questionnaire for Patients With Chest Pain (Cleary 1991) are examples of instruments suited to specific problems. Based on this entire body of generic work and specific applications, Hamilton and Granger, supported by federal funding and encouraged by national rehabilitation associations, sought to develop standardized scales to measure medical rehabilitation outcomes, burden and costs of care that could be used with facility in rehabilitation wards and hospitals. The resulting Functional Independence Measure (FIM) (Keith et al. 1987) is an 18-item index which measures self care, sphincter control, mobility, locomotion, communication and social cognition which is being used in conjunction with financial data to produce a uniform data set in over 300 rehabilitation facilities in 12 countries (Laughlin et al. 1992).

In a similar integrative effort in the mental health arena, Becker et al. (1993) have designed a new instrument for measuring quality of life in persons with severe and persistent mental illness (QLI-MH). The QLI-MH gathers demographic information and assesses nine different domains of quality of life including: (1) satisfaction levels with different aspects of quality of life, (2) occupational activities, (3) psychological wellbeing, (4) physical health, (5) social relations, (6) economics, (7) activities of daily living, (8) symptoms, and (9) goal attainment. Individual scores are calculated for each domain and an overall QOL score is obtained by summing values across domains. The instrument is used to establish individual and groups norms for those with severe and persistent mental illness and to monitor patients' responses to treatment both in institutions and in the community.

While all of this work was useful in developing an approach to subjective health assessment and health-related quality of life, there was a simultaneous pressing need to construct valid and reliable instruments that provided a generic profile of health status applicable to the general public as well as to those with disabilities and special conditions. Three widely used instruments were developed in the 1970s with this purpose in mind, the Sickness Impact Profile (SIP) (Bergner et al. 1981), Nottingham Health Profile (NHP) (Hunt et al. 1980, 1985, 1986) and the McMaster Health Index Questionnaire (MHIQ) (Chambers et al. 1976). These related instruments were constructed as behaviourally based measures of health status. The SIP was developed to provide a indicator of perceived health status over time and across groups. The MHIQ, like the SIP, incorporated measures of self-perceived physical, social and emotional functioning to determine health status. The NHP also taps what individuals are feeling when they experience different levels of illness and activity limitation.

This body of work, including numerous related scales and studies based on them, currently defines the field of subjective health assessment and health-related quality of life. So far, theoretical and conceptual work has lagged behind instrument construction and validation. As a consequence, different domains and dimensions of subjective health assessment have been identified and measured but considerable effort remains to situate this work in a meaningful theoretical framework. On the positive side, the recent theory building of Antonovsky (1993) in elaborating his Sense of Coherence theory to explain resiliency and ability to deal with stressful events and the integrative work of Stewart & Ware (1992) and Patrick & Erickson (1993) are encouraging signs that these efforts are under way.

The validity and reliability of subjective health assessment

While subjective health assessment is being viewed as increasingly important, conceptual, design and measurement problems abound. How does an interviewer persuade respondents to provide an accurate assessment of their perceived health conditions in a way that reflects true, personal experience and in a manner that is not unique to that individual? Such measurement problems connected with subjectively perceived health status raise issues of validity and reliability. Questions of internal validity ask: did the instrument measure what it purports to measure?

External validity refers to the generalizability of the instrument and results. Reliability addresses the question: Is this assessment accurate across time and contexts? These are important issues, for health interventions based on subjective health assessments are likely to have limited effectiveness unless the service provider knows the patients' perceptions and preferences at the time of the intervention and can generalize to a larger group. Furthermore, interventions can lose their impact if patients change their perceptions and preferences during the course of treatment and the intervention is not appropriately adjusted. The researcher and clinician, then, either have to be reasonably certain that individuals will not change their perceptions or they must do periodic re-assessments and modify interventions accordingly.

The task before clinicians and researchers alike is to design instruments to measure subjective health status with validity and reliability, which can be used on different populations groups and over time. Similar problems of validity and reliability pertain to the sampling procedures and study designs employed to assess the effect of treatment interventions on health outcomes (Mohr 1992). While the problems are considerable (Heyink 1990, Robinson 1990), initial steps have been made to develop and fruitfully apply subjective measures in health services research and clinical practice.

Subjective health assessment scales are evaluated in terms of their content, criterion and construct validity, for if these instruments do not have acceptable validity, they cannot be used in outcomes research and clinical practice. Content validity refers to the representativeness or sampling adequacy of the content purportedly measured by the scale; in this case health-related quality of life. Much of the work on subjective health assessment instruments has focused on defining content domains and dimensions. While there has been some disagreement about which constituent domains to include in scales and represent in the definition of health-related quality of life, there is a growing consensus about the critical elements and even how they are to be measured. Elaboration and modification of existing scales and field testing is leading to better instruments.

The key issues are the domains included in the instruments and the context in which they are intended to be used. Some broad-ranging scales are intended to provide a general health profile; others are disease or institution specific. Some scales are for children, others for adults or the elderly. Some scales are designed to measure health status in the general population; others on sick populations. To be effective, the instruments selected must fit the population, context and purposes of the particular study or clinical application. The content validity of the major health-related quality of life instruments is good but often not all domains are covered. Also care is to be exercised in extending their use into different populations without extensive pretesting and piloting.

Criterion validity concerns whether or not the variable can be measured with accuracy. Psychometricians are interested in a scale's concurrent and predictive validity when they consider criterion validity. Concurrent validity asks if one scale can be substituted for another in a given situation. If both scales are administered to subjects at the same time, they should be highly correlated. The Katz (Katz et al. 1963) and Barthel (Mahoney & Barthel 1965) scales of Activities of Daily Living, for example, should be highly correlated. Predictive validity concerns the scale's ability to predict from levels of physical function to mobility in the community. The commonly used measures of physical function and mobility have moderate to high criterion-related validity (Albrecht & Higgins 1977). The global health profile scales like SIP, NHP, and MOS generally have acceptable criterion validity but the results differ by audience and use (Bowling 1991, Stewart & Ware 1992).

Construct validity refers to the power, adequacy and precision of the constructs that theoretically underpin the actual measurement instruments. Construct validity attends to the theoretical adequacy of the model being employed and allows the researcher to test alternative explanations and to construct causal arguments from the results of studies. If a scale has good construct validity, then other constructs and theories ought not to be able to explain the results with equal facility. Cook and Campbell (1979) suggest that this is the most important type of validity for it allows science to accumulate evidence, build powerful explanations of behavioural outcomes and rule out spurious arguments. Unfortunately, these are also the areas where subjective health assessment and health-related quality of life research are weak. Experts working in health-related quality of life can make significant advances if they pay more attention to construct validity, theory building and controlling for confounding variables.

Further threats to validity are posed by the use of proxy measures to obtain quality of life information on individuals who are unable to communicate, are cognitively impaired or are too weak to undergo the rigours of an interview. In these instances health care providers and/or family and friends are asked to complete the instruments for the patient/respondent. Such a technique is particularly important in studies of older people who are likely to experience prolonged chronic illnesses and subsequent ongoing supportive relationships with medical care providers, family and friends. Proxy measures in these instances permit the study of those recovering from strokes and the frail elderly. Studies of older adults show that physicians and other proxy respondents tend to underestimate patients' quality of life (Rothman et al. 1991). When judgements on aspects of quality of life are compared between patients and their proxy respondents, the proxy respondents tend to agree with the patients in the more directly observable domains like physical functioning, activities of daily living and cognition. They are more likely to disagree with patients in the assessment of pain, feelings of anxiety, depression, perceptions of general health, changes in health status and self care deficits (Magaziner et al. 1988, Epstein et al. 1989).

These findings present a dilemma: the use of proxy respondents permits for the study of populations where quality of life is a major issue, yet these measures are not always valid and reliable. Such situations call for more methodological work to improve accuracy under these conditions. In the meantime, validity can be enhanced by asking patients to nominate their own proxies. Research shows that proxies selected in this fashion tend to report more reliably (Bassett et al. 1990). In addition, proxies will respond more accurately if they are given clear instructions. They can also be asked to rate the perceived accuracy of their responses. Finally, investigators should avoid proxy estimations of highly subjective domains like pain, depression and affective feelings until more precision can be guaranteed.

Instrument reliability ensures that the scale will consistently obtain the same results when administered multiple times or in different circumstances. Scale reliability and validity ensure that changes in scores indicate changes in attitudes, perceptions or behaviour. Reliability is ascertained by using multiple forms of the same instrument, split half and test-retest techniques and correlating the results to see if both forms or randomly selected sets of items correlate highly. The Cronbach's alpha coefficients are reasonably good for most of these subjective health assessment instruments but the results are often influenced by population sampled, context and purpose to which the results will be put (Bowling 1991, Stewart & Ware 1992). Cronbach's alpha is a commonly employed measure of internal reliability for multi-item summated indices which is calculated by averaging all the possible split-half reliability coefficients (Cronbach 1951, Aday 1989).

Additional problems with interpreting results from these instruments involve the scoring of the scales and use of the results. Most instruments like the SIP, FIM, MOS and QLI-MH contain subscales measuring separate domains. Respondents can be given a score on each of the quality of life dimensions to distinguish them from other individuals and groups. Moreover, a summary total score can be constructed by aggregating the scores of each dimension to indicate a general health related quality of life score. Such an approach is conceptually appealing but analytically difficult. Each of the dimensions like physical functioning and emotions are conceptually distinct and probably multidimensional in themselves. A simple aggregation procedure to achieve a summary health-related quality of life indicator poses serious problems of identifying, weighting and interpreting the component elements in each of the subscales as well as the over-all score. Consequently, a simple comparison of total scores to determine relative quality of life differences between individuals and populations can be misleading, unless one examines the constitutive elements and distributional patterns of the subscales in each instrument. For these reasons Cox et al. (1992) suggest that simple aggregated summary scores should not be used in comparing quality of life across individuals and groups.

Closing the gaps between theory and practice

While problems abound in the design and use of subjective health assessment instruments, corrective actions and inventive techniques can be employed to refine conceptual models and employ results in a thoughtful manner. As the field matures in theory and measurement, investigators can best proceed by exercising caution and sound judgement in designing and executing studies and interpreting results. Theories undergirding health-related quality of life and subjective health assessment studies can be improved by building on recent advances in our understanding of wellness, women's health, the life course, social and cultural contexts and social networks.

An emphasis on well rôles focuses attention on preventive actions and an integration of health and lifestyle (Glik & Kronnenfeld 1989). In terms of quality of life this reorientation highlights healthful activities and the social-psychological consequences of feeling healthy and in a "life balance" (Antonovsky 1993). The new international initiatives to undertake massive epidemiological and intervention studies on women's health recognize that women's physiology and health experiences are different from those of men. Therefore, theories of health-related quality of life should take such differences into account in study design and interpretation (Riessman 1983, Muller 1990). Research on health, illness and disability across the life course indicates that life course experiences and ageing are not the same as chronological age (Albrecht & Levy 1991). Subjective health experiences are most likely to differ according to one's position in the life course. As a consequence, subjective health assessment would be more informative if it were sensitive to life course context.

Social and cultural contexts also affect health and one's perceptions of illness. When conducting field research on infant and maternal health in the Kenyan highlands in 1971, a researcher reports that he noticed that his African interpreter had cold sweats and the "shakes" in the cot next to him as the team was going to bed (Albrecht 1973). He remarked to the experienced Kenyan physician, "I think that this man has malaria." The doctor replied, "Everyone who lives in this area has malaria. No problem." Recently in Russia the same researcher was interviewing sex workers in an HIV/AIDS related study. One sex worker reported that she did not use condoms with customers, if they paid her enough. When asked why, she responded, "Work is work. I need the money and I am not going to get AIDS from wealthy Western businessmen." The point is that people interpret disease, risk and health in terms of their own social and cultural situations. These factors are critical in the design of subjective health experience instruments and studies, but have received insufficient attention to date.

Social networks are important in subjective health assessment and health-related quality of life studies because the network defines people's comparison and support group (Wilson 1993). Health and illness are social in nature. The care and support of those who are ill or disabled is a demanding social activity. To understand subjective health experiences, people's social resources and relationships must be identified and their perceptions of this support known. If these related bodies of theory and research are incorporated into the conceptual foundations and design of health-related quality of life studies, they will improve the body of work.

In terms of methods, a closer integration of ethnography, qualitative and quantitative techniques will provide greater depth and perspective to the work (Brewer & Hunter 1989). In a quality of life study on paraplegics, for example, investigators struggled to explain why some patients sampled in comprehensive medical rehabilitation facilities made no improvement in function and even refused therapy. None of the variables in the regression analysis would explain these behaviours. Finally, out of frustration the investigators identified those patients who made no progress and interviewed them (Granger et al. 1979). When asked why they were not making progress in their rehabilitation programme, one patient answered, "If I get better, I will have to return to work. I am 58, tired and disabled. I want to receive disability benefits and go home." Another responded, "It's too much work. I will not go through that pain and suffering and still be disabled. Leave me to my wheelchair." Another remarked, "I believe in Jesus. When Jesus calls me out of my chair, I will get up and walk. I do not believe in doctors." These experiences underline the importance of doing ethnographies and qualitative interviews before quantitative instruments are finalized. Pilot studies and pretests will also uncover material that markedly improves the quality of the research. Certainly such information is invaluable in interpreting outcomes and rethinking interventions.

Conclusion

This paper provides an orientation to subjective health assessment by situating the field in an historical context, pointing out the progress that has been made in measuring health-related quality of life and applying the results, indicating methodological and theoretical problems that may be encountered and suggesting approaches to address those difficulties. Subjective health assessment opens an entire new area of research and aspect of clinical practice that is crucial as physicians focus on problem-oriented and patient-centred medical care. This approach switches attention from medicine to the larger issues of health and wellness. The context also changes from that of medical institutions to the home and community. If patients' perceptions and feelings are taken into account in health care decision making, patients will become empowered and more actively engaged in the maintenance and management of their own health. This perspective also fits with a more market driven and competitive health care delivery environment where consumer needs and preferences will be important considerations in the allocation of scarce resources.

Subjective health assessment represents a value reorientation in research and clinical practice. It is an essential foundation for bringing civility and humanity back into medicine by taking patients' perceptions, feelings and problem contexts into account in understanding need and delivering care. For these reasons the future of subjective health assessment is bright. At the same time, it is important to realize the limitations of current theory and methods. The challenge, then, is to move the field to its potential.

CHAPTER 3

Applications of health status measures

Ray Fitzpatrick

Introduction

In the short period of twenty years or so that health status measures have been available, a very wide range of applications have been suggested. It is increasingly clear that the very different contexts in which they may be used may require very different measurement properties and practical features for an instrument to operate effectively. This chapter examines four quite distinct applications. At one extreme it is suggested that health status instruments have a very practical rôle in helping health professionals to gain a full picture of their patients, or health authorities to identify patterns of need in local populations. At the other extreme are the various research uses of health status measures as indicators of outcome in clinical trials or cost–utility studies.

Individual patient care

The most commonly considered applications of health status measures are those that are more research-oriented, for example clinical trials or evaluation studies where health status measures are used to assess outcomes of health care interventions for scientific purposes. However it is also argued that they may play as important a rôle in improving the health care of individual patients.

Two related but distinct clinical applications can be identified. They may serve as screening devices, where the primary objective is to identify problems that the health professional might fail to recognize. Or they may serve as mechanisms to monitor the course of patients' progress over time, make decisions about treatment and assess subsequent therapeutic impact. These two uses are related in that, as is argued below, screening is only worthwhile if it results in some kind of improved care. The use of health status measures as a screening instrument requires that patients complete such instruments when seeking health care and that the information thus obtained is then made available to the health professional to assist his or her decision-making. Some studies have demonstrated that psychiatric screening questionnaires can be useful in increasing doctors' awareness of the extent and nature of psychological problems in their patients (Johnstone & Goldberg 1976). Clinicians are unaware of a substantial proportion of such problems in their patients and increasing their awareness may improve the overall quality of health care. However other evidence is less encouraging about the benefits of psychiatric screening. In one trial patients attending a number of doctors in a primary care setting completed a psychiatric screening questionnaire (Hoeper et al. 1984). In the experimental group patients' screening data were given to their doctor whereas for the control group this information was withheld. Physicians were then required to make psychological assessments of all patients in a separate medical record. Unfortunately there were no significant differences in their accuracy of judgement of psychological wellbeing in experimental compared with control patients, so that, by inference screening had not improved diagnostic judgement.

The logic behind psychiatric screening instruments is just as applicable to the broader range of problems identified by health status instruments given the evidence that health professionals are unaware of many of their patients' problems in this broader sense (Sprangers & Aaronson 1992). Similar studies have now been carried out to evaluate the results of providing clinicians with data from health status instruments used to screen attending patients. For example, several studies have examined whether clinicians find the information offered by health status measures useful or informative. Some studies have obtained encouraging results with the majority of clinicians finding such additional data helpful in allowing a more comprehensive assessment of the patient and improving communication between doctor and patient (Young & Chamberlain 1987, Kazis et al. 1990a, Rubenstein et al. 1989).

Requirements of a screening test

It is important to recognize that, as with other forms of screening, such as radiological or biochemical tests, so the use of health status measures to screen patients can only be justified if the screening instrument is accurate, results in more effective treatment than would otherwise be the case and does so with a favourable ratio of costs to benefits (Mant & Fowler 1990). The accuracy of a screening test is determined by its sensitivity, specificity and predictive value. Sensitivity is the proportion of individuals with a disease that a test detects. Specificity is the proportion of individuals without the disease so identified by the test. Predictive value is probably the criterion of most relevance to a health professional using a screening test in clinical practice. It is concerned with the proportion of all those predicted by the test as having the disease who prove to have the disease. All of these parameters are harder to determine with health status measures than many conventional screening tests, because the entity being screened is less clearly defined and less precisely measured. There will be less clarity regarding "real" levels of disability or social isolation in a patient group than regarding presence or absence of cancer or diabetes. The assessment of health status measures has generally been examined in terms of validity rather than through the framework of screening tests. Health status measures are therefore assessed by whether they appear adequately to address an underlying construct rather than in terms of precise estimation of numbers of "false alarms" (false positives) or "false reassurance" (false negatives).

For some more "objective" aspects of health status there are ways of examining health status measures as if they were screening tests. Studies have established that self-reported aspects of disability and physical function can agree very closely with standard clinical tests of performance or observers' judgements (Sullivan et al. 1987). However, even with more physical aspects of health status, absence of close agreement with external criteria may not be evidence of a flawed test if the purpose of the test is actually to assess subjective difficulty or concern about physical function rather than physical function *per se*. Similarly, there are a number of studies that have demonstrated the ability of health status measures to predict other health outcomes such as subsequent deterioration in health or mortality (Kazis et al. 1990b, Reuben et al. 1992).

The second criterion for the evaluation of a screening test is whether it results in effective treatment of the problem screened. It is unethical to screen for health care problems for which there is no effective care available for those positively identified. This is an important perspective for evaluating health status instruments in the context of individual patient care because it underlines the need to demonstrate some net beneficial outcome to patients. It raises the second issue identified earlier: what rôle health status reports play in the subsequent management and outcomes of health care problems. It is possible that information from health status instruments may influence the processes of care, so that, for example, health professionals make different clinical decisions as a result of the additional information. However, if the criteria of screening tests are still applied, far more important would be evidence that the use of health status instruments in health care improved outcomes. A few studies have begun to examine impact of health status instruments on outcomes. Thus Kazis and colleagues (1990a) conducted a trial to examine the benefits gained by informing clinicians of their patients' health status scores. Patients all had a diagnosis of rheumatoid arthritis and the health status instrument used varied, either the Arthritis Impact Measurement Scale (AIMS) (Meenan et al. 1980) or the Modified Health Assessment Questionnaire (MHAQ) (Pincus et al. 1983). Patients in one group (the so-called "experimental group") completed health status instruments which were sent to clinicians on a quarterly basis over a year. An "attention placebo" group completed the instruments quarterly but data were not passed on to their doctor. A control group only completed instruments at the beginning and end of the study. There were no detectable differences between groups at the end of the year in process variables such as changes in medication or referrals to other agencies. Nor were any differences obtained in terms of outcomes such as patient satisfaction or change in health status. A similarly designed study examined the benefits of using the Functional Status Questionnaire (FSQ) (Jette et al. 1986) to screen patients with various disabilities four times over one year (Rubenstein et al. 1989). Again no differences were found between experimental and control groups in either processes of care such as treatment decisions or outcomes in terms of health status.

The third and last issue in assessing the value of health status instruments in individual patient care is that of costs in relation to benefits. As has been argued, benefits in terms of health gain have not yet been clearly demonstrated. One benefit that warrants further investigation is the evidence that patients welcome the opportunity of giving clinicians evidence about their health status completed in questionnaires and consider the information important for clinicians to know (Nelson et al. 1990). At one extreme there is a danger of such uses in a clinical context being a "marketing ploy" in which health status screening is used to demonstrate the institution's *perceived* customer orientation but not to inform the provision of care. Other costs that need to be considered are, less the raw materials of self-completed questionnaires which tend to be inexpensive and more the costs of processing, storing, retrieving and interpreting patient-based data which may well be substantial.

Overall clinicians have not rushed to add health status instruments to their clinical practice. Many clinicians currently find the information conveyed via health status instruments irrelevant to clinical decisions, both time-consuming and difficult to interpret and too cumbersome to integrate into familiar clinical routines (Deyo & Patrick 1989). There is still substantial work to be done in identifying the appropriate timing of feedback from instruments to clinicians (Greenfield & Nelson 1992). These various practical considerations have led many to conclude that only the shorter and simpler forms of instruments, such as the Dartmouth COOP charts (Beaufait et al. 1992), will ever stand a chance of becoming accepted parts of clinical practice. Brevity and economy have to be traded off against precision and comprehensiveness in the clinical context. Some current evidence suggests that shorter instruments do not necessarily lose very much of the information conveyed by longer versions (Katz et al. 1992).

Population measures

Increasingly health care systems attempt to match the provision of health care to the needs of populations. Indeed purchasing authorities in the NHS are required to do so. Existing measures of need, largely in the form of socio-demographic variables and mortality data do not provide information that is sufficiently specific to inform decisions about resource allocation. It is often argued that health status instruments provide an important new source of information about perceived health need (Hunt et al. 1985). Their advantages include the fact that they are relatively inexpensive to administer (via the mail), compared with conventional epidemiological measures that tend to require clinical expertise, and also they assess the "consumer's" perspective more directly than more medically driven approaches. Bodies such as the UK Healthy Cities Network have advocated the development and use of a "Quality of Health Life Indicator" for such reasons (Thunhurst & MacFarlane 1992). Studies are beginning to appear that use health status instruments to assess and compare the health needs of different local populations (Curtis 1987). It is suggested that health status instruments may not only provide consumer-oriented data of health needs in order to maximize the appropriate provision of health care; they also offer the possibility of population-based bench-marks against which to judge the impact of health care provision over time (Ware et al. 1981).

To date the best case that has been made for the use of health status measures in informing the planning of health care for local populations has been in providing additional evidence for inequalities in health status between particular social groups. Thus evidence has accumulated of inequalities in health status by social class, gender, ethnicity and employment status (Ahmad et al. 1989, Jenkinson et al. 1993a, 1993b). Such evidence can be used as "ammunition" to support broader approaches to health policy and resource allocation at the local level. However, the more problematic application of health status instruments is in informing decisions about resource allocation for specific interventions and services. It has to be questioned whether health status instruments provide sufficiently precise information for such purposes (Donovan et al. 1993).

Predictive value in a population context

Some problems are more technical and methodological. Thus one of the more widely cited health status instruments – the Nottingham Health Profile (NHP) (Hunt et al. 1986) – has a basic flaw as a population instrument, namely that the modal response in general populations is zero (i.e. very favourable) (Kind & Carr-Hill 1987, Brazier et al. 1992). With such a distribution of scores, it is unlikely to provide useful discrimination between levels and types of health need. More generally there is likely to be a problem with the predictive value of health status instruments in general populations. The predictive value of a screening instrument may be high in a hospital context with a high prevalence of underlying disease but low in a general population.

A more fundamental objection to their application as a measure of health need in local populations, is that the evidence generated is of fairly non-specific symptoms and concerns very broadly defined problems such as pain, mobility and social function. While the meaning of such problems may be clear in the context of a clinical trial or intervention with a particular patient group with identified health problems, in the context of a population survey they may offer little or no evidence of need for particular health care interventions (Frankel 1992). It has been argued that more ethnographic methods of obtaining more detailed and sensitive health perceptions are needed instead of standardized health status instruments in order to provide more informative data about health needs (Donovan et al. 1993). However the case for such alternative methods is even less convincing at present. At least it is conceivable in principle, that standardized quantified measures of fairly precise problems such as difficulties in using transport or being able to reach shops could provide feasible targets against which to assess progress, particularly if measured repeatedly over time in clearly identified sub-groups, such as individuals with particular disabilities or chronic illnesses.

Clinical trials

The most successful applications of health status instruments have been their use as outcome measures in clinical trials and research evaluations of health interventions. It is increasingly recognized that many of the diagnostic and therapeutic technologies used in health care have not been demonstrated to be effective by the most exacting of methods (Department of Health 1992). In particular it is argued that health technologies need to be subjected to randomized controlled trials in which patients are randomly allocated either to receive a treatment that is the subject of investigation or to a control group where they receive either a placebo or a comparable active treatment. This methodology provides the most precise estimate of benefits to patients from an intervention. For some interventions mortality may be the most relevant measure of outcome. However an enormous range of medical and surgical interventions are partly or largely intended to have beneficial effects on aspects of patients' wellbeing other than survival. Thus, for example, joint replacement surgery is intended to decrease pain, improve mobility and expand the range of daily activities that an individual can perform. Similarly pharmacological or psychotherapeutic management of a patient with schizophrenia is intended to improve a wide range of aspects of the personal and social functioning not only of the patient but of his or her family. In all such cases the need to provide measures of the impact of treatment on many aspects of patients' wellbeing indicates an important contribution to be made by health status instruments.

There are also many health care interventions which may have a mixture of beneficial and harmful effects on the patient. Thus a number of drugs used in the treatment of cancer may prolong survival but also are sufficiently toxic that they can have a range of harmful effects on the patient such as nausea or depression (Byrne 1992). Similarly a wide range of drugs have been developed with beneficial effects of lowering blood pressure, thereby reducing risks of stroke in individuals. At the same time they may also have negative effects on the patient's mood, social and sexual functioning (Croog et al. 1986). In this area of health care, health status instruments have a vital rôle to play in providing measures of the extent of harmful effects that may have to be traded off against benefits.

Health status measures thus have an important rôle in addressing quite specific questions regarding impact upon patients' wellbeing of particular drugs or forms of surgery. However as health care has become more technical and dependent on increasingly complex forms of organization and delivery, so it is also possible to address issues regarding the effects on health status of alternative forms of delivering health care. The randomized trial provides a widely applicable format for examining questions such as whether particular treatments are more effectively delivered on an inpatient or outpatient basis; whether teamwork has more favourable effects on care of chronic illness; and whether patient-centred forms of conducting consultations improve outcomes. In all of these examples the trial-format of research design can be used to examine alternative ways of providing care, and health status instruments may be used as the primary measures of outcome. Even broader and more economic issues concerning health care can be turned into scientific questions by this methodology. Probably the most well known application of health status measures in a trial was the RAND Health Insurance experiment to examine the health and economic consequences of "cost-sharing" (i.e. requiring patients to pay directly a fee at the time of using the health service) (Ware et al. 1986). Patients were randomly allocated to various forms of cost-sharing and impact on health status was measured by a variety of conventional medical measures such as blood pressure, cholesterol and mortality, as well as a sophisticated battery of questionnaire-based health status measures.

Health status measures offer a particularly powerful method of evaluating the benefits or costs of health care in the context of clinical trials. A randomized trial can result in quite clear interpretations of health status scores provided that the trial is well designed (Cox et al. 1992). Full randomization has the consequence that differences in health status can be clearly attributed to aspects of the intervention rather than pre-existing differences between patients. Patients are carefully followed up over time to assess changes in baseline health status scores and care must be taken to take account of any loss to follow-up that might bias results (for example, patients with poorer health status in one treatment-arm of a trial may refuse to take part in the trial). Patients recruited to trials are normally quite homogenous in terms of their health problems and diagnoses so that changes in health status arising from the trial can be clearly interpreted in the light of other knowledge about the patients, their health problems and the possible mechanisms of action of the intervention that they have received. Most importantly, unlike other applications of health status measures, such as cost–utility analyses (described below), different dimensions or aspects of health status, such as pain and psychological mood are measured and analyzed separately so that specific and possibly contrary trends between dimensions can be detected. For clinical trials it is important to know that, for example, a drug has beneficial effects on pain but harmful effects on mood, so that there is little point in averaging out or combining such effects across dimensions.

Appropriate measures for clinical trials

Health status measures provide a highly informative method of measuring appropriate outcomes in trials. Yet the majority of randomized clinical trials still either fail altogether to use health status measures, or use measures that are untested or inappropriate. Thus a review of clinical trials published in major medical journals such as *New England Journal of Medicine* or *Annals of Internal Medicine* found that in only 10 out of 55 trials was an appropriate health status measure used despite such measures being vital or important to the appraisal of the intervention in the opinion of the reviewers (Guyatt et al. 1989). A similar review of publications in oncology and cardiology examined scientific publications of trials with the term "quality of life" in the title, abstract or key words. The authors concluded that in only one-third of publications were appropriate measures of the term actually used (Schumacher et al. 1991). Other reviews have come to similar conclusions (Najman & Levine 1981). In the main, trials that ought to be using appropriately validated health status instruments either fail to use any measure or use measures that only address a partial aspect of health status, or are *ad hoc* and have not been tested for basic measurement properties such as reliability and validity.

Whereas the most important requirement of health status instruments, when used to screen for undetected problems, may be described as their predictive value, in the context of clinical trials the measurement property that is of most concern is "responsiveness", that is the capacity of an instrument to detect significant changes over time in health status, even if those changes are rather small. Instruments that have been shown to be valid measures of aspects of health status may still not be particularly sensitive to important changes within individuals over time (Guyatt et al. 1992). This may arise for a variety of reasons. Thus categories of an instrument may be too broad to detect subtle changes in the patient. Despite experiencing real changes in, for example pain, the respondent has to select the same broad category to describe himself on two occasions. Another problem can arise from too many items of an instrument not being relevant to the treatment of a trial or the particular patient group so that the few items that may be responsive to changes experienced by a patient group are swamped by the numbers of items that are static.

The solution to maximizing responsiveness is to select items that are particularly relevant to the intervention being examined. This may not always be possible as, in some cases, trials are conducted in which there are few prior hypotheses about possible areas of positive or negative health consequences and very broad measures of health status are therefore used to detect unanticipated effects. An additional suggestion is to maximize the gradations of measurement for important dimensions so that even modest changes can be registered by the respondent. Also items should be included that are frequent and salient for the majority of patients since clinically meaningful changes are more likely to be found in trials for important problems than for dimensions of health status that few patients experience as a difficulty (Guyatt et al. 1993). Responsiveness of instruments also needs to be examined statistically in slightly different ways from those used to test validity. In particular, agreement with change scores for other relevant variables becomes more important than static, cross-sectional correlations (Fitzpatrick et al. 1993).

Health status in cost–utility analysis

A quite distinct application of health status measures is in the context of the economic appraisal of health care interventions. It is increasingly argued that, given limited health care budgets and the enormous actual and potential demands for health care faced by such budgets, authorities responsible for the allocation of resources should attempt to maximize the amount of health gain that can be obtained from use of health care resources (Williams 1985). In order to do so, health authorities require information about two distinct aspects of all the different medical, surgical and other treatments provided, that is information about the costs associated with different interventions and about the benefits from interventions in terms of health gain. These two components provide information that would permit comparisons between health interventions in terms of health benefits as a ratio of costs. Advocates of this perspective argue that it is in the interests of health authorities to allocate resources to those treatments that achieve the greatest gain for a given unit of resource.

The full set of calculations involved in such analyses is beyond the scope of this chapter. However, an understanding of the measurement of health gain used in such economic appraisals is important. It is postulated that any health care intervention may be considered to have, overall, a given net benefit in terms of health, compared with notional or actual patients with the same condition(s) who do not receive the intervention. This benefit arising from the treatment may be considered to have two components – survival, or added years of life, and an adjustment to the added years derived from the health states expressed as quality of life. The two components combined, usually expressed as "quality adjusted life years gained" (QALYS) represent in one figure the impact of an intervention upon a single overall index of health (Williams & Kind 1992).

A method is therefore required that can capture and express the "quality of life" component of QALYs. This requires the capacity to do two related but distinct tasks. First, one needs a reasonably comprehensive system for describing a full range of health states, so that, for example, within the descriptive system, effects of such disparate interventions as psychotherapy, orthopaedic surgery and renal dialysis can be expressed uniformly. Secondly, a method is required of attaching values to the set of descriptions of health states. This second requirement arises from the need to express in a uniform manner the overall benefits, or, in economists' terms, "utilities" derived from interventions. A global value is then obtained for any given combination of survival and quality of life resulting from the intervention. Finally, data on costs of interventions are combined with data on benefits expressed as quality adjusted life years gained to derive a single summary expression of costs per quality adjusted life year gained, which will be the unit of comparison between interventions.

The first step in the derivation of a set of utilities expressing the values attached to benefits of health care is therefore a set of descriptions of a range of health states. One of the most widely cited sets of descriptions is the classification of illness states by Rosser (Rosser & Kind 1978). This system employs a two dimensional matrix in which health states are considered to be a combination of a particular degree of disability (with a range from "no disability" to "unconscious") and of distress (with a range from "no distress" to "severe distress"). It has been acknowledged that this is not a particularly comprehensive system to describe health states and Rosser added a third dimension, physical discomfort (Rosser et al. 1992). In order to be more comprehensive Rosser and her group have developed an instrument, the Index of Health Related Quality of Life, with 44 scales to assess more specific components that contribute to distress, disability and discomfort.

The initially simple Rosser Index, therefore, has been developed in the direction of greater comprehensiveness and specificity in the new index. However the practical cost of this is clearly the complexity of the instrument required to assess health states, which now runs to 225 descriptive statements that may be made of a patient. This may jeopardize the feasibility of the instrument. Another approach to health status assessment has attempted to remain brief and easy to complete, while addressing a broad array of health states. The Euroqol instrument requires respondents to rate health on six dimensions (mobility, self care, main activity, social relationships, pain, mood) each of which has two or three simple alternative options (e.g. for mood options are "not anxious or depressed" versus "anxious or depressed") (Williams & Kind 1992).

The main requirements of such systems is that they be applicable to the widest range of health problems, in view of the fact that they will be used ultimately in cost–utility analyses to compare effects on health of, for example, coronary artery bypass surgery and psychogeriatric services. If a descriptive system were less sensitive to health problems in a particular area, then results would less accurately reflect cost–benefit relations for interventions in that area and would ultimately distort resource allocation. It is conceivable that some of the very broad categories of the Euroqol (Euroqol Group 1990), for example, "depressed or anxious" versus "not depressed or anxious" do not permit very precise degrees of distinction to be made between levels of psychological ill health. Not only do such general measures need to be sensitive to the widest range of health states, also, just as in the clinical trials context discussed earlier, they must be maximally sensitive to changes over time. There is evidence, for example that the early version of the Rosser Index is not particularly responsive in at least some areas of health (Donaldson et al. 1988).

Utilities

As described above, there is a second component to the measurement of health status as applied to cost–utility analysis, namely the calculation of values or utilities associated with health states. Values assigned to varying degrees of disability, pain distress etc. are obtained by judgements of panels in experiments. A variety of techniques have been developed for this purpose, most commonly: standard gamble, time trade-off, category scaling, magnitude estimation, equivalence and willingness to pay (Richardson 1992). They have in common that they elicit from experimental, hypothetical tasks judgements regarding the relative undesirability of different health states. These utilities are the global figure used to adjust survival rates in relation to interventions.

A number of problems arise in relation to the derivation of utilities. Different experimental tasks produce somewhat different valuations of health states. There is some evidence of disagreement between individuals' valuations; with some disagreement related to the individual's background and previous experience of illness (Froberg & Kane 1989). There is also evidence that individuals do not make well informed judgements when asked to imagine the experience of hypothetical illness states (Kahneman & Varey 1991). It is particularly hard to imagine the benefits of therapies in terms of transition from one health state, prior to treatment, to another (after treatment).

There are broader ethical and policy problems that arise from the application of such methods to cost–utility analysis and hence resource allocation, which are beyond the scope of a book on health status measurement and are discussed elsewhere (Carr-Hill 1989). There are enormous practical and logistic problems arising from lack of any real data for most interventions. The philosophical underpinning of the whole approach is utilitarian – the greatest good for the greatest number of people. However this runs up against equally appealing principles such as egalitarianism – that every individual is entitled to some health care (Potts 1992). Some groups such as the elderly may be systematically disadvantaged by current versions of QALYs (Grimley Evans 1992). In principle it should be possible to disentangle moral and ethical issues from problems of measurement but, as in other areas of social science, the substantive problems become too closely identified with matters of value.

Applications in the sociology of illness

Finally it needs to be recognized that apart from the applied uses of health status measures so far discussed, there is potential for them to contribute to our basic sociological understanding of health problems. With the array of measures now available, a number of core issues can be addressed. Relationships between health status and wellbeing are not straightforward, with individuals often making adjustments to illness that are remarkable to the observer without experience of illness (Bury 1991). Health status measures should enable us to examine more precisely to identify the psychosocial processes involved. Conversely we should begin to understand more clearly the specific demands of illness that do reduce wellbeing (Devins et al. 1993). Another field of application would be the examination of social differences in health status arising from social class, ethnicity and gender (MacIntyre 1986a). Health status measures may also allow a more empirical examination of the factors in addition to health care that contribute to health. To date such debates have largely been confined to evidence from mortality statistics, and health status measures offer an alternative means of examining the contributions of other social, behavioural and environmental factors to health.

CHAPTER 4

Measuring changes in health status

Sue Ziebland

Introduction

The increasing use of health status questionnaires in the monitoring of outcomes has highlighted sensitivity to change over time, or "responsiveness", as a vital characteristic (Guyatt et al. 1987, Fitzpatrick et al. 1992). Not all of the questionnaires which are in current use were originally designed to tap this feature, having been intended to provide "snapshot" descriptions of the health of a population. However, since there are relatively few applications which do not involve the reliable assessment of change (Jenkinson et al. 1993b), there remains concern about the ability of some measures to respond to changes that are of clinical and subjective relevance.

One longitudinal study of the relative sensitivity to change of a number of health status measures used in rheumatoid arthritis (Fitzpatrick et al. 1993) revealed considerable between-questionnaire variations in the impression of improvement, stability and deterioration gained from a group of one hundred patients at a rheumatology clinic. A battery of disease specific, generic and conventional clinical measures were repeated at three-monthly intervals. Effect sizes were calculated according to the method recommended by Kazis et al. (1989), as the difference between the mean scores of two completions, divided by the standard deviation at time one. This calculation was made in order to compare the extent and direction of the changes that were indicated by the different instruments. At follow-up the patients described their progress by completing a five point transition index concerning their improvement, stability or deterioration since the last visit. The magnitude of the differences between the instruments was such that, among the third of the patients who characterized themselves as having improved (either greatly or slightly) over a three-month period, the change scores on one questionnaire would indicate substantial and significant improvement, while another questionnaire would show no changes and a third would show only slight changes. Given the variability between instruments, it is clear that in circumstances where only one questionnaire is used, misleading conclusions could be drawn. On the other hand, researchers who favour the use of several measures could be engaging in a somewhat baffling practice if a battery of indicators provides inconsistent, or downright contradictory, evidence. The discovery of such variability is therefore important and clearly worth pursuing.

The object of this chapter is twofold. In the first section methods of assessing change in health status will be described and discussed. In the second part some of the aspects of research design and questionnaire selection which may hamper responsiveness will be addressed.

Methods of assessing change

Sensitivity to change is an indispensable characteristic of any health status instrument that is to be used as an outcome measure. To be of any practical value, it is also important that the meaning of changes in the scores are simple to interpret. Treatment trials should state at the outset what level of change will be considered clinically significant, given the nature of the intervention.

Changes from baseline

Although the health status at the end of a study may be seen as the outcome of interest, it will often be the magnitude of the changes that more appropriately reflects the treatment effect. One of the advantages of basing analysis on change scores is that they remove any differences between the groups with respect to pre-treatment levels of the outcome variable (Altman 1991). However, one should beware of ceiling and floor effects whereby patients who score at the extreme end of a questionnaire are unable to register improvement (or deterioration) in later assessments (Bindman et al. 1990).

Effect sizes

Lydick and Epstein (1993) have identified effect sizes as the most commonly cited of the distribution-based interpretations of change scores. The most commonly used method of calculating an effect size is to divide the mean change between baseline and follow-up, by the baseline standard deviation. Kazis et al. (1989) have demonstrated the use of effect sizes in identifying changes which are clinically meaningful in preference to the rather less discriminating criteria of statistical significance. An effect size of 1.00 is equivalent to a change of one standard deviation in the sample. As a bench-mark for assessing the relative magnitude of a change, Cohen (1977) identified an effect size of 0.20 as small, of 0.40 as moderate and of 0.80 as large. It has been suggested that effect sizes may not be the most appropriate method for comparing the sensitivity to change of different instruments, because they do not incorporate the response variance. Standardized response means (SRMs) may be more appropriate for this purpose. SRMs are equal to the mean change in score divided by the standard deviation of individuals' changes in scores (Katz et al. 1992).

Global transition judgements

Global rating scales require the respondent to describe their state of health through answering just one question, such as "Would you describe your health as very good, good, fair, poor or very poor?" There is evidence for the value of such simple global ratings (see, for example, Gough et al. 1983, and the chapter by Rowan in this text). One of their most useful features is that units of change have the undeniable benefit of clarity. Similarly, changes over time can be successfully measured by simply asking the patient to make a direct judgement about the extent of improvement or deterioration (as in "much better", "slightly better", "the same", "slightly worse", "much worse"). The use of transition items has been validated against other criteria (Pincus et al. 1989), and it has been demonstrated that they do not seem to be contaminated by the patient's mood (Fitzpatrick 1993). Although global transition items, such as those asking about overall changes in health, may be used to assess the outcome of a specific intervention (Doll et al. 1992) there is a danger in more complex conditions of obscuring conflicting aspects of the course of an illness, whereby one aspect may have improved while another has deteriorated. It is also possible that global transition judgements may be dominated by variations in a particular symptom, such as pain.

Transition scales

Multiple-item transition scales enable patients to rate the extent to which they have improved or deteriorated on a number of key variables, thereby allowing for the possibility that not all functions and symptoms will respond in the same manner. This method may also be considered where baseline measures are not plausible, such as in intensive care or accident and emergency outcomes research, although the respondent's reference point for the comparison would need careful definition.

There is evidence that patients can express the course of their health more accurately through these direct judgements, than may be picked up by repeated use of the baseline questionnaire. In a study of patients with rheumatoid arthritis, a comparison was made of two approaches to representing changes measured by the Health Assessment Questionnaire (HAQ) (Ziebland et al. 1992b). The HAQ includes eight sections which cover various aspects of daily life, such as reaching, getting in and out of bed, dressing and climbing stairs. Respondents are invited to describe the amount of difficulty they have been experiencing with each task during the past week, selecting from "without difficulty", "with some difficulty", "with much difficulty", or "unable to do". Three months after the first administration the HAQ was administered again, but in addition to the conventional computation of the change score between two assessments, respondents were also invited to complete an eight item transition index where specific tasks were indicated as "more difficult", "less difficult" or "stable" since the last interview (see Figure 4.1.).

Tables 4.1 and 4.2 show the quite striking differences between the two methods when correlations with other indicators of change in disease activity are examined.

The use of a small set of transition items to measure changes as a follow-up to a full baseline assessment of health appears to have much to recommend it: it is quick to complete, requires minimal scoring and provides the opportunity for an unequivocal representation of changes which are of relevance to the patient.

Compared with three months ago how difficult is it now (this week) to . . . (For each item respondents choose from "less difficult", "the same", "more difficult")
Dress yourself, including tying shoelaces and doing buttons? (dressing)   Get in and out of bed? (rising)   Lift a cup or glass to your mouth? (eating)   Walk outdoors on flat ground? (walking)   Wash and dry your entire body? (hygiene)   Bend down to pick up clothing from the floor? (reach)   Turn taps on and off? (grip)   Get in and out of the car? (activities)

Figure 4.1 Items on the HAQ transitional scales.

Table 4.1 Correlation coefficients (Pearson) for clinical variable change scores with transitional HAQ (*p < 0.01, **p < 0.001).

Transition items on MHAQ	Ritchie Index	Grip	Pain	Morning stiffness	ESR	Hb
Dressing	−0.16	0.03	0.02	0.11	0.11	−0.17
Rising	0.04	−0.10	0.13	0.00	0.16	−0.06
Eating	−0.07	−0.03	0.05	0.07	0.02	−0.16
Walking	0.12	−0.20	0.16	0.12	0.12	−0.06
Hygiene	0.03	−0.16	0.07	0.10	0.25	−0.09
Reach	0.25	−0.29*	0.16	0.15	0.32*	−0.11
Grip	0.16	−0.23	0.12	−0.06	−0.03	0.17
Activities	0.12	−0.34**	0.09	0.12	0.17	−0.03

Table 4.2 Correlation coefficients (Pearson) for clinical variable change scores with HAQ change score (*p < 0.01, **p < 0.001).

Transition items on MHAQ	Ritchie Index	Grip	Pain	Morning stiffness	ESR	Hb
Dressing	0.35**	−0.30*	0.44**	0.33**	0.48**	−0.36**
Rising	0.37**	−0.35**	0.43**	0.30*	0.46**	−0.33**
Eating	0.37**	−0.34**	0.37**	0.25	0.39**	−0.10
Walking	0.37**	−0.30*	0.49**	0.34**	0.39**	−0.23
Hygiene	0.35**	−0.38**	0.38**	0.31**	0.52**	−0.25
Reach	0.27*	−0.37**	0.32*	0.27*	0.39**	−0.24
Grip	0.39**	−0.40**	0.42**	0.32**	0.37**	−0.19
Activities	0.31*	−0.30*	0.34**	0.27*	0.39**	−0.37**

Research design and questionnaire selection

Ware (1981) draws attention to the main criteria against which generic health status instruments should be selected, and stresses the careful attention which must be paid to item content. A number of guides to the field of health measurement have become available in recent years (Wilkin et al. 1992, 1993, Bowling 1991) and advise users of health status questionnaires to choose carefully when making a selection, ensuring that appropriate domains are included. Thus, if a treatment is designed to alleviate pain and encourage mobility, then these will be vital inclusions in the measure. Although there are a number of disease specific questionnaires available, it should not be assumed that such instruments will automatically include all of the dimensions which are most germane to people with the condition, nor that they will necessarily include the most appropriate indicators of the outcomes of a particular treatment. The purpose of this section of the chapter will be to demonstrate that it is necessary to look beyond the titles of the domains to the actual content, where it will be shown that rather different aspects of (ill) health are being tapped by different questionnaires, despite the uniformity which is suggested by domain titles.

Tacit models of disability

Examination of the content of the most widely used health status questionnaires reveals the existence of four distinct models of disability which are used in the measurement of physical function, mobility and activities of daily living. Described as the functional, subjective distress, comparative and dependence models (Ziebland et al. 1993), these can be shown to influence both the respondents' baseline scores and the responsiveness of these scores to subsequent changes in health. The effects which the models have on the ability to discern differences in health status have specific implications for research design, some of which will be discussed here.

The functional model

Items which are based on the functional model concern disqualification from the performance of a function or activity. Responses are invariably dichotomous, with respondents simply affirming those statements

47

which apply to them. Examples are:

> "I'm unable to walk at all." (Nottingham Health Profile (NHP),
> Hunt et al. 1985)
>
> "I do not walk at all." (Functional Limitations Profile (FLP),
> Patrick and Peach 1989)
>
> "I do not keep my balance." (FLP)
>
> "Can you walk a block or more?" (RAND Functional Status
> Indexes (RAND FSI), Stewart et al. 1978)

Some of the benefits of the functional model are the simplicity of the items and the fact that responses are relatively uncontroversial, thus inter-rater agreement could be anticipated to be fairly high. There is also the opportunity for addressing a wider range of functions than would be possible in most conventional clinical settings, thus allowing an assessment of the impact of a condition on the patient's normal life. However, the fact that a patient is unable to express modifications such as the degree of difficulty or pain which they experience, or the amount of time it takes to perform the task, means that this model may lack discrimination at any but the most extreme levels of function. Similarly, repeated assessments are likely to be insensitive to any but the most dramatic changes in function. Hence a patient whose mobility is steadily deteriorating will not affirm an item until there is total exclusion from the performance in question.

The subjective distress model

This model overcomes some of the inherent problems of the functional model by focusing on the degree of difficulty which the respondent experiences. Although the responses may still be of a dichotomous nature the statement will include a qualifying adverb, "easily", for example, or provide a scale for responses such as the HAQ categories of "no difficulty", "some difficulty", "much difficulty", "unable to do". Examples of this model are:

> "Do you have any trouble either walking several blocks or climbing a few flights of stairs because of your health?" (Arthritis Impact Measurement Scales (AIMS), Meenan et al. 1980).
>
> "Can you easily button articles of clothing?" (AIMS).
>
> "I find it hard to stand for long," (NHP).
>
> "Today, do you (or would you) have any physical difficulty at all with cooking?" (McMaster Health Index Questionnaire (MHIQ), Chambers et al. 1982).

The greater subjectivity of the assessments are likely to lead to less inter-rater reliability, although such reliability has been shown to be high on the HAQ (Fries et al. 1982). This model certainly allows the respondent to describe their performance with more latitude than the functional model; however, positive changes will still have to be of a fairly striking nature before a respondent is able to record that they have become able to open a jar of food "easily", as one of the AIMS items requires.

The comparative model

Two variants of the comparative model can be identified. The first of these involves normative comparisons, whereby the respondent considers their own health in relation to other people:

> "I seem to get sick a little easier than other people," (Short-Form 36 Health Survey Questionnaire (SF-36), Ware & Sherbourne 1992).

> "I am as healthy as anyone I know," (SF-36).

Comparisons with others may be a useful indication of the respondent's perception of the handicapping aspects of their condition. There is concern that these assessments will be heavily influenced by the respondent's age and social circumstances and the associated difficulties of symptom attribution, and thus be too inconsistent for most purposes. The designers of the London Handicap Scale (Harwood et al. in press) have tried to overcome this problem by specifying that questions should be answered in comparison with others of the same age, sex and background whose "health is good". Without such instructions, it is probable that judgements made within a hospital setting, where the existence of people with more severe disabilities may be very evident, will differ from those conducted in other settings, with different reference groups.

The other frequently used comparisons are those which require the respondent to express their current health state compared with their "usual" or former condition. Such habitual comparisons include:

> "I am cutting down on some of my usual physical recreation or more active pastimes," (FLP).

> "I can work for as long as I usually do," (Self-rating pain and distress scale (PAD scale), Zung 1983).

> "I walk shorter distances or often stop for a rest," (FLP).

Questions based on this model may be very useful for assessing the impact of a temporary illness, or a period of flare-up within a longer term condition. The process of gradual adjustment which often takes place to accommodate the effects of a chronic condition may, however, render some surprisingly modest scores on such items. An example of this may be found in a study where people who had RA for 12 years or more scored significantly more favourably on a scale composed of habitual comparisons (the "recreations and pastimes" domain of the FLP) than those with a less longstanding illness, despite having more severe levels of disease according to a battery of clinical variables and the HAQ (Ziebland et al. 1993).

The dependence model

A number of questionnaires include items concerning the respondent's use of aids or personal assistance, which may be taken to indicate the extent of a disability. Sometimes questions about assistance will feature explicitly, while the instructions for the HAQ state that scores should be increased if help is used. The following are examples of the dependence model:

"I need help to walk about outside," (NHP).

"Are you unable to walk unless you are assisted by another person or by a cane, crutches, artificial limbs, or braces?" (AIMS).

"When you travel around your community does someone have to assist you because of your health?" (AIMS).

"I only use stairs with a physical aid, for example, a handrail, or stick or crutches," (FLP).

"I only get dressed with someone's help," (FLP).

Clearly there are some types of assessments where it is useful to record the amount of personal help which is needed, and the growing rehabilitation industry (Albrecht 1992) can provide aids which enable many people with disabilities to live independent lives. However, when this model is applied in health status measurement, the assumption that access to aids and personal assistance is any sort of surrogate for a measure of severity belies the reality that people's ability and willingness to make use of help is a characteristic with enormous individual variation.

A concentration on the use of assistance may obscure considerable changes over time. An example is the HAQ, where scores increase to 2 ("much difficulty") on any section where help of a personal or mechanical nature is used for the listed activities. As a result, if this questionnaire were to be used to assess the outcomes of an occupational therapy service, any distribution of appropriate aids to people whose original scores were less than "2", would register as an apparent deterioration at follow-up. Clearly, this would be in contradiction to the beneficial effects of the service.

Circumstances in which the questionnaire is completed

In any research it is important to address features of the design which might systematically bias the results. Responses to any standardized questionnaire will be subject to a degree of background noise, as people make sense of the questions and provide accounts in a diverse and sometimes splendidly idiosyncratic manner, despite the apparent limitations of the closed response set (Donovan et al. 1993). It is customarily assumed that any such "noise" will be of insufficient decibels to deafen the data-analysis and that a large enough sample will cancel out any irregularities of response. However, there are circumstances in health measurement in which responses are highly likely to be systematically confounded by routine factors. An example is when the respondent completes the questionnaire from a hospital bed (Jenkinson et al. 1993c).

There are potentially many reasons why being in hospital could influence a patient's self-reported health status. One could anticipate elevated anxiety and depression scores, and a probable decline in rôle performance coupled with access to adapted facilities which could improve the ability to perform some self care. On the other hand, any impact which hospitalization may have on rest, sleep disturbance and social activities is probably too subject to individual variation to predict. Bardsley et al. (1992) measured the effect of hospitalization on responses to the NHP and reported that it seemed unaffected by completion in this location. However, in a study of patients with RA, the 36% of respondents who were originally recruited when inpatients had significantly elevated scores on just one measure of mobility, the FLP mobility scale. This was despite having very similar scores on other domains and on clinical tests (Jenkinson et al. 1993c). It has been suggested that it is not necessary to take recourse to sophisticated analysis to understand why this should have occurred, given that the following statements contribute 56% of the score of the FLP mobility scale and that the FLP instructs respondents to affirm those statements which apply to them "today" and which are due to their health (Ziebland et al. 1992a):

"I only get about in one building."
"I stay in one room."

"I stay in bed more."

"I stay in bed most of the time."

"I do not use public transport now."

"I do not go into the shopping centre."

There are a number of research designs which require at least one completion of a health status measure while the patient is in hospital. If domains which are influenced by hospital setting are utilized as outcome measures, then restricted physical function may be assumed where the immediate cause is actually the inevitable restrictions of the hospital ward. This would clearly have a confounding effect on the interpretation of scores which appear to improve dramatically upon the respondent's release from hospital.

Conclusion

The development of a range of generic and disease specific self completion questionnaires for measuring patients' health has coincided with an increasing recognition that physicians do not always make accurate assessments of their patients' health-related quality of life (Slevin et al. 1988, Calkins et al. 1991). Calls for patient assessed measures to be used as a routine tool of clinical practice (Wolfe and Pincus 1991) and requirements for providers of treatment to demonstrate the outcome of their interventions, combine to make the increased use of health status questionnaires all but inevitable. In many ways it is a development which should be welcomed, for it provides the patient with an opportunity to express the impact of treatments on the physical, emotional, symptomatic and social components of health. However, despite much apparent uniformity in the components of questionnaires, it cannot be assumed that similarly titled dimensions are actually measuring the same thing.

Many of the observations which have been made in this chapter will be familiar to researchers who have conducted interviews using health status questionnaires, yet in large studies the people who collect the data (and are thus attuned to some of the problems of the methodology) are often not the people who do the analysis, nor those who are responsible for choosing the instruments to be used in the study. As a result of this, some of the difficulties inherent in the approach may never get addressed. However, when health status measures are used routinely by clinicians to assess the outcome of their work they are likely to be closely involved in all stages of the administration and analysis of the data and so will be aware of results which seem to be counter-intuitive. If discrepancies are large enough to present clearly improving patients as stable, it will not be surprising if the clinician loses faith in patient-based assessment. It is therefore important that the selection of the original questionnaire is made with great care, that wider aspects of the research methods, such as place of completion, are considered in detail, and that the method of assessing changes encourages the patient to report in a manner which is intelligible both to themselves and to those involved in their care.

CHAPTER 5

Global questions and scores

Kathy Rowan

Introduction

The growing interest in the measurement of health status from the perspective of the patient has led to a large number of increasingly sophisticated instruments being developed for this purpose. However despite
this, and perhaps in part because of this, health status measures are not
routinely used by providers of health care in the assessment of patients.
This may be attributed to lack of knowledge of the existence of such
measures, scepticism by clinicians of the usefulness of such measures,
and also concern as to the amount of time and resources needed to
routinely administer and score such questionnaires. This chapter will
address the issue as to whether single item global health questions can
provide valid and useful information, without consuming the amount of
time and resources needed for more elaborate measures.

It will be clear to the reader, both from the other chapters in this book
and from other relevant literature (McDowell & Newell 1987, Bowling
1991, Wilkin et al. 1992), that there are many valid and reliable measures
available for assessing the health status of patients. For the most part,
measures contain a series of questions designed to assess one or more
dimensions of a patient's health state. Health status measures may be
generic (a measure designed to be of general applicability for use with
any illness or population group) or specific (intended for specific illness
groups).

Health status profiles provide a series of scores, one for each dimension of a patient's health status. Each individual score represents a combination of the responses to a number of questions for each dimension of

health state included in the measure. Health status profiles may include such dimensions (or domains) as general health, physical functioning, social functioning and ability to sleep, although dimensions assessed on such measures vary. Examples of such profiles are the Sickness Impact Profile (SIP) (Bergner et al. 1981), the Short-Form 36 General Health Survey Questionnaire (SF-36) (Ware & Sherbourne 1992) and the Nottingham Health Profile (NHP) (Hunt et al. 1986).

Single index measures

Whereas health status profiles provide a series of scores, single index measures summarize these as a single index figure of health status. Thus the responses to all questions on every dimension of health state contribute to the overall score. Examples of such index measures are the Nottingham Health Profile Distress Index (McKenna et al. 1993), the Quality of Well Being Index (Kaplan and Anderson 1988), the Quality of Life Index (QL-Index) (Spitzer et al. 1981) and the Euroqol (Euroqol 1990).

Over the last few decades a great many measures of health status have been developed, validated and tested for reliability. However, while questionnaires have proliferated, the search for the ideal measure (short, cheap, simple to use, psychometrically sound, measuring the important aspects of subjective health status and sensitive to change) has continued. Kane (1987) summed up the requirements for the ideal measure as the need for "the clinical equivalent of the Swiss army knife, something small and easily taken into the field with enough blades and attachments to fit any number of circumstances that may arise". One of the major problems with health status profiles and single index measures is that they usually include a large number of questions which potentially limit their practical use. The length of questionnaires raises the criticism that they are too time-consuming both to complete and to score for routine use in the assessment of patients.

If providers of health care are to be expected to measure the subjective health status of their patients routinely, the measures they use must balance brevity and practicality with validity. Without doubt, the shortest and simplest assessment is a single question requiring an overall description of health status, yet uncertainties exist as to the adequacy of such evaluations. This chapter addresses the issue as to whether a global score derived from a single, global question provides valid information. To answer this, it is necessary to establish the validity of the data generated from global questions.

Do single, global questions provide valid information?

A global score is one derived from a response to a single global question. For example, a global score for overall health status might be based on a global question such as "In general, how would you rate your overall health?" with a choice of answers from "excellent" through "very good", "good" and "fair" to "poor". By designating a score to each category (for example, one for "excellent" through to five for "poor") a global score is provided.

While global questions may refer to the general health of a person, an alternative is to anchor questions to a particular dimension of health, such as emotional state, or to a specific health concern, such as the overall bothersomeness of a particular set of symptoms. Global questions ask either about current health status or, as transition global questions, about current health status relative to a previous occasion, for example before surgery or since the last assessment.

In an attempt to evaluate the validity of global questions, comparisons have been made between global scores and scores derived from more complex measures such as health status profiles and single index measures. For example, Chipperfield & Marks (1992), using data from the Bloomsbury and Islington Health and Lifestyle Survey found a strong association between increasing Nottingham Health Profile (NHP) scores (i.e. reporting more health-related problems) and worsening self-rated general health, using the single, global question "Over the last 12 months, would you say your health has on the whole been good, fairly good, or not good?" Mean NHP scores between the "good", "fairly good" and "not good" categories, grouped by response to the global question, were significantly different from each other for both sexes and for all six dimensions of the NHP. Similarly, Rowan (1992), using data on over 3000 patients who had undergone intensive care treatment in the UK approximately six months earlier, also found a strong association between increasing NHP score and worsening self-rated general health, using answers to three different global questions. The questions were:

(a) Overall health: "How would you describe your health at present (Very good/Good/Fair/Poor/Very poor)?" (see Fig. 5.1)
(b) Limitations: "Is your health status (Good health, no limitation in daily activities/Some limitations in daily activity but able to live an independent life/ Severe limitations in daily activities, not able to live an independent life)?" (see Fig. 5.2)
(c) Comparative health: "Compared with other people of your age and sex, would you say your health is (Better than average/Average/Worse than average)?" (see Fig. 5.3).

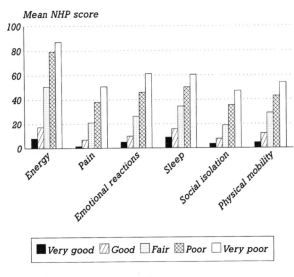

Figure 5.1 NHP scores broken down by overall health, for respondents who received intensive care treatment six months earlier (see text).

Global questions have also been used to determine the criterion validity of longer form measures. Criterion validity refers to the extent to which results on one measure are associated with results from a separate measure, the latter being taken to be the criterion variable or "gold standard". Doll et al. (1993), took a global health question as the "criterion" variable against which dimensions of the NHP were judged. They found a strong association between increasing NHP score and worsening self-rated general health, using answers to the single, global question

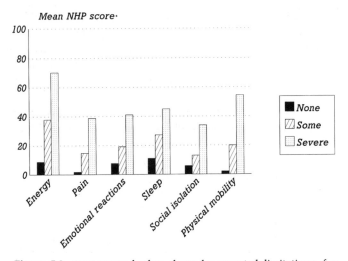

Figure 5.2 NHP scores broken down by reported limitations, for respondents who received intensive care treatment six months earlier (see text).

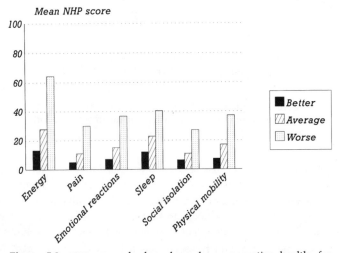

Figure 5.3 NHP scores broken down by comparative health, for respondents who received intensive care treatment six months earlier (see text).

"Overall, how would you rate your health over the past month? (excellent/very good/good/fair/poor)". They gained data from 388 men in hospital awaiting surgery for benign prostatic hypertrophy and reported clear linear trends of increasing group mean NHP scores with worsening self-rated general health. These results were statistically significant for all six of the dimensions (energy, pain, social isolation, emotional reactions, sleep and physical mobility) of the NHP.

As part of the development of a short health status measure, Ware et al. (1992a) observed a substantial degree of correlation between responses to each of six, single global questions, one for each dimension of health status, and the combined responses to multiple questions for the same dimensions in the full length version of the Medical Outcomes Study (MOS) questionnaire. Correlations between responses to each of the global questions and the combined responses to multiple questions were high and statistically significant: for physical functioning (10 questions in MOS) 0.74, social functioning (4 questions in MOS) 0.83, rôle functioning (10 questions in MOS) 0.71, bodily pain (6 questions in MOS) 0.71, psychological distress (18 questions in MOS) 0.77, and general health (7 questions in MOS) 0.76. In addition, within each of the five response categories of the global question (excellent/very good/good/fair/poor), the mean scores for the seven question, general health dimension from the full-length MOS questionnaire were remarkably similar for two large but different samples (Table 5.1).

Table 5.1 Response to a global question on general health and group mean scores for general health on the full-length MOS questionnaire (modified from Ware et al. 1992).

Global question response	Mean general health score (MOS questionnaire)	
	Sample 1	Sample 2
Excellent	87.9	86.9
Very good	75.5	75.4
Good	57.6	55.9
Fair	30.0	30.6
Poor	10.8	10.8

Note: Global question, "In general, would you say your health is excellent/very good/good/fair/poor?" Higher scores indicate better health status (max = 100).

Jenkinson et al. (1993c) reported similar findings for the SF-36 dimensions when broken down by the single, global question "In general, would you say your health is excellent/very good/good/fair/poor?". These findings are discussed in greater depth in Chapter 7.

The results of global questions have also been compared with results gained from longer instruments in which the items all contribute to an overall "index figure". Spitzer et al. (1981), as part of the development and validity testing of a five item, single index measure known as the QL-index, found high correlations between results from this measure and a single global question answered on a visual analogue scale. Similarly, Gough et al. (1983), using data on 100 patients with advanced metastatic cancer, found highly significant correlations between responses (on a visual analogue scale) to a single global question "How would you rate your general feeling of wellbeing today?" and two valid, reliable, single index measures, the QL-index (both interviewer and self-administered) and a modified LASA-21 (Linear Analogue Self-Assessment) questionnaire (Baum et al. 1980).

Global items have also been used in the assessment of change over time. The ability of an instrument to measure change over time is important in the evaluation of treatment regimes and interventions. It is important that measures can detect clinically important changes. It is possible to evaluate change by asking questions of health status at two points in time and calculating the difference between scores, or by asking patients to directly assess change since some specified point in time. Such "transition items" can take the form of global assessments of health status. For example, Ziebland et al. (1992b), using data from 100 patients with rheumatoid arthritis, found a high level of association with scores for a series of six standard rheumatological measures assessing disease activity and the global question "Thinking of any overall effects your arthritis may have on you: how would you describe yourself compared with the last time I interviewed you (three months ago). Are you: much better, slightly better, the same, slightly worse or much worse?", asked at the second assessment.

Doll et al. (1993), using data from 388 men in hospital awaiting surgery for benign prostatic hypertrophy and data collected 12 months after the surgery, reported the association between change in NHP scores and response to a transition global question relating to perceived overall change in health status; "Overall, how do you rate how you feel now compared to before your prostate operation. Do you feel: Much better

now/A little better now/About the same/A little worse/Much worse?".
The worse patients reported they felt after surgery compared with before
surgery, the smaller was the reduction in NHP score. Linear trends were
observed for all dimensions of the NHP, although non-significant for
physical mobility. Figure 5.4. summarizes the findings, broken down by
patients claiming they felt better, the same or worse.

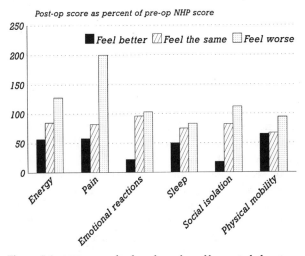

Figure 5.4 NHP scores broken down by self-reported change
in health status since surgery for benign prostatic hypertrophy
(see text).

From these examples, it is apparent that global single item measures
of health state can provide information that, at the very least, is consistent with more complex methods of assessment. Global general health
questions provide an overall health summary that is supported from
data gained from longer instruments. It is possible to disaggregate the
components of overall health into single questions concerning specific
aspects of health. When careful consideration is given both to the selection of such questions and to the scores assigned to the scale of responses, substantial correspondence between scores derived from single,
global questions and scores derived from multiple questions, for the
same dimension of health status, are observed (Ware et al. 1992a). Such
results have led some authors to conclude that single, global questions
are valid to use in the assessment of patients (Gough et al. 1983). Others

have questioned whether there is any added value in administering more complex questionnaires, especially with reference to the significant savings in research costs in using single, global questions (Chipperfield & Marks 1992). While in instances where brevity is essential global questions may be appropriate instruments, the high correlation of global scores with other more complex measures does not justify the wholesale rejection of profiles or single indices. This chapter will now turn to the possible benefits and limitations of the various ways health status may be evaluated.

Benefits and limitations of global questions

The use of global questions to assess health status is not new. The General Household Survey – an annual survey of a stratified random sample of about 15,000 households in the UK – poses two global questions about health. One seeks to determine the prevalence of household members whose normal activities have been limited by longstanding illness during the preceding two weeks. The other focuses on the recent incidence of acute illnesses. Similarly, the National Center for Health Statistics in the USA asks respondents to rate their general health using a single, global question.

The benefits associated with the use of single, global questions mainly relate to their practical application. They are short and quick, both to administer and to score. They are simple to answer and there is no need for specially trained personnel to administer, record and interpret their results. Compared with more complex measures, they are cheaper to use. The clarity and brevity of single global questions may produce higher response rates (Rowan 1992), perhaps indicating greater acceptability to the respondent. Missing data (for example, where less than 100% of the items in a scale are answered) is a perennial research problem for which some imaginative remedies have been suggested – this dilemma is undeniably simplified through the use of global questions.

If the benefits which are accrued through the use of global questions are primarily practical, the limitations tend to be related to the sensitivity of the data. A loss of information is one of the obvious trade-offs in using a single question to measure health status. In their work on patients with rheumatoid arthritis, Ziebland et al. (1992b) observed that "the global transition item . . . obscures a feature of [rheumatoid arthritis] activity whereby some functions may improve while others are in decline".

Global questions share many of their other limitations with the more complex health status measures. These may include a tendency to skewed responses and the possibility of "floor" and "ceiling" effects which have also been observed with the NHP (Kind & Carr-Hill 1987, Brazier et al. 1992) and the short-form instruments developed from the RAND studies (Bindman et al. 1990, Ware et al. 1993). Floor and ceiling effects, sometimes referred to as "end" effects, refer to the tendency of questionnaires to either (1) pick up only the very severe end of ill health, thereby tending to under-represent the extent of ill health in a given sample, or to be (2) highly sensitive to minor levels of ill health, thereby tending to over-represent the ill health of a given sample. Thus, on the one hand, one possible impact of these characteristics is that any but the most dramatic differences between respondents are likely to be obscured. On the other hand, where improvements or deteriorations within an individual are modest, they may not be apparent longitudinally. In questionnaires containing small numbers of items, or global questions, there is a greater likelihood of such effects.

In summary, the research question or clinical interest is paramount when choosing a health status measure. Among the most important criteria are the resources available, the context in which the measurement is to be made and the level of accuracy required. Furthermore, if it is predictable that responses to a complex health status measure will, for the purposes of analysis, be re-coded into broad categories, the substitution of a simpler measure at the outset may be preferable.

Current developments relevant to global questions

Recent developments have been focused on measures incorporating a single, global question for each dimension of health status included in the measure. There have been a number of developments in this area. This section will review three of these developments namely the Short-Form 6 (SF-6), the COOP charts, and the Modified Health Assessment Questionnaire (MHAQ). These questionnaires provide a profile of responses, yet are simple to complete and score, and thus may have both advantages of brevity and comprehensiveness.

The SF-6 Health Survey Questionnaire

Ware et al. (1992a), in the pursuit of brevity and comprehensiveness, have developed a questionnaire covering six dimensions of health status (physical functioning, social functioning, rôle functioning, bodily pain, psychological distress and general health perceptions) using a single, global question to cover each dimension. They have reported on the logic underlying the selection of each of the global questions for each dimension and preliminary results of its construct and discriminant validity have found it to be appropriate for group-level analyses. The measure needs further evaluation in terms of its precision, namely its ability to detect small differences in health status between groups and its use in monitoring changes in health status for individual patients over time.

COOP charts

These charts have been developed by the Dartmouth Primary Care Co-operative Information Project (Nelson et al. 1990, Beaufait et al. 1992, Wasson et al. 1992, Bruusgaard et al. 1993). Pictorial charts measure health status for nine dimensions (physical condition, emotional condition, daily work, social activities, pain, change in condition, overall condition, social support and quality of life). Each has a simply worded question with five response categories and each response category is linked to a drawing intended to represent that health state. A copy of the charts is reproduced at the end of this chapter. Unlike many other measures, the COOP charts have been specifically developed for use in routine clinical practice. The COOP charts have been assessed for validity and reliability and have compared well with longer measures. While reducing respondent burden substantially when compared to long-form measures utilized in the Medical Outcomes Study, the loss in precision when compared to the longer measures was minor (McHorney et al. 1992). In America research with the charts has so far been encouraging, with both clinicians and patients claiming that the inclusion of this questionnaire in the medical interview has improved the consultation and provided both sides with important information (Kraus 1991). The charts need further evaluation in terms of their use outside America and outside routine clinical practice for which they were designed. In addition, the designers have suggested that the content and style of pictures and the administration may influence patient response: further research is required on this. The charts also need further evaluation in terms of their precision, namely the ability to detect small differences in health status between groups, their use in monitoring changes in health status for individual patients over time and their sensitivity to detect clinically important change.

The Modified Health Assessment Questionnaire

Pincus et al. (1983) developed the Modified Health Assessment Questionnaire (MHAQ), an adapted version of the HAQ, a 20-item, eight dimension, health status profile used for measuring health status of patients with rheumatoid arthritis. MHAQ contains eight, transition global questions, one for each of the eight dimensions of health status (dressing, rising, eating, walking, hygiene, reach, grip and activities) included in the original HAQ questionnaire. The questions are reproduced in Chapter 4 of this text. Each question asks patients to assess whether they are the same, improved or worse for each dimension compared with a specific previous occasion. In the original study, the transition questions were asked retrospectively, without an anchor point, to assess changes in difficulty over the six months before the interview, in order to predict the level of satisfaction with the ability to perform tasks. In a study comparing the original HAQ, completed on two occasions three months apart, with the MHAQ transition questions, completed only on the second occasion, it was found that the transition questions of the MHAQ were more strongly related to other rheumatological changes, measured as change scores for a series of six standard, rheumatological measures assessing disease activity, than were change scores (the difference between the score at one assessment and the next) from the HAQ. MHAQ also showed advantage over a single, global transition question which, though correlated with the rheumatological measures, obscured a function of rheumatoid arthritic disease whereby some functions may improve while others are in decline (Ziebland 1992b). A more detailed account of this study appears in Chapter 4 of this text. The results of the study could add support to the view that not only can single items provide data economically, but they can also do so accurately. Furthermore, considerable economy is achieved in the case where single items are used to assess changes over time after treatment (thereby removing the need for assessments to be made prior to and after treatment). The MHAQ is, of course, a disease specific measure and more research is, as yet, needed to determine whether similar results could be obtained using a measure comprised of "generic single item change scores".

Conclusion

The search for the optimal measure – simple, cheap, short, acceptable to both users and respondents, valid, reliable and sensitive to change – continues. However, if one considers that the components that comprise a good health state are multiple and include such dimensions as physical, social and emotional health, and that for different conditions different dimensions of health status are important, the following two conclusions are apparent. The first is that no universal method, whether a complex measure or a single, global question, will be appropriate in all settings. The second is that it is undeniable that single, global questions will always provide less explanatory power than more comprehensive measures.

The rudimentary nature of global scores may limit their usefulness for detecting small to moderate differences between groups and for monitoring changes in health for individual patients over time. However, there is some evidence that transitional global questions may more accurately reflect changes over time than change scores derived from repeated applications of more complex measures. It is not argued here that global questions, either current or transitional, should totally replace such measures. However, it may be worth considering the proposal by Ziebland et al. (1992b) that baseline administration of a health status questionnaire could be followed by subsequent assessment using transitional global questions covering specific functions or dimensions, rather than repeated use of the original instrument. Such assessments may provide a clearer reflection of the patient's experience, be quicker to administer and to score and provide results that are more meaningful to clinicians than numerical change scores derived from a complex health status measure.

In this chapter, the contribution of global questions for the requirements of research and for routine clinical practice has been considered. Single, global questions are both simple and economical as well as useful, although this chapter is not intending to imply that this is all we should have. There is evidence that in some cases a single global question may be as informative as longer, more complex measures which consume more resources as a consequence of their administration. Amongst these resources is the, too often overlooked, goodwill of the respondent, although the impact on clinical time is also clearly crucial. Many of the problems inherent in global questions apply to more complex measures: the challenges of sensitivity, validity and reliability, for example, are common to the whole field of health status measurement.

In summary, there are trade-offs which are being well documented in the research literature so that future researchers may select the most appropriate instruments for their purposes. There may be no one, perfect, health status measure reducible to an ultimate, indisputable single index figure. Improvements within the arsenal of research instruments mean that, if research questions are clearly defined and if appropriate instruments are chosen (be they health status profiles, single index measures or global questions), the prospects for conducting truly informative research into the impact of health interventions have never been better.

PHYSICAL FITNESS

During the past 4 weeks . . .
What was the hardest physical activity
you could do for at least 2 minutes ?

Very heavy, (for example) •Run, fast pace •Carry a heavy load upstairs or uphill (25 lbs/10 kgs)		**1**
Heavy, (for example) •Jog, slow pace •Climb stairs or a hill moderate pace		**2**
Moderate, (for example) •Walk, fast pace •Carry a heavy load on level ground (25 lbs/10 kgs)		**3**
Light, (for example) •Walk, medium pace •Carry light load on level ground (10 lbs/5kgs)		**4**
Very light, (for example) •Walk, slow pace •Wash dishes		**5**

1

FEELINGS

During the past 4 weeks . . .
   How much have you been bothered by
   emotional problems such as feeling anxious,
   depressed, irritable or downhearted and blue ?

Not at all		**1**
Slightly		**2**
Moderately		**3**
Quite a bit		**4**
Extremely		**5**

9/88

2

DAILY ACTIVITIES

During the past 4 weeks . . .

How much difficulty have you had doing your usual activities or task, both inside and outside the house because of your physical and emotional health ?

No difficulty at all		**1**
A little bit of difficulty		**2**
Some difficulty		**3**
Much difficulty		**4**
Could not do		**5**

3

SOCIAL ACTIVITIES

During the past 4 weeks . . .
   Has your physical and emotional health limited
   your social activities with family, friends,
   neighbors or groups ?

Not at all		1
Slightly		2
Moderately		3
Quite a bit		4
Extremely		5

4

PAIN

During the past 4 weeks . . .
How much bodily pain have you
generally had ?

No pain		**1**
Very mild pain		**2**
Mild pain		**3**
Moderate pain		**4**
Severe pain		**5**

5

CHANGE IN HEALTH

How would you rate your overall health
now compared to 4 weeks ago ?

Much better	▲ ▲ ++	1
A little better	▲ +	2
About the same	◀ ▶ =	3
A little worse	▼ —	4
Much worse	▼ ▼ ——	5

6

OVERALL HEALTH

During the past 4 weeks . . .
  How would you rate your health in general ?

Excellent		1
Very good		2
Good		3
Fair		4
Poor		5

7

SOCIAL SUPPORT

During the past 4 weeks . . .

Was someone available to help you if you
needed and wanted help? For example if you

— felt very nervous, lonely, or blue
— got sick and had to stay in bed
— needed someone to talk to
— needed help with daily chores
— needed help just taking care of yourself

Yes, as much as I wanted		1
Yes, quite a bit		2
Yes, some		3
Yes, a little		4
No, not at all		5

8

QUALITY OF LIFE

How have things been going for you during
the past 4 weeks?

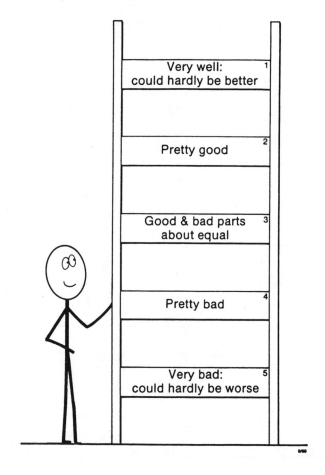

9

CHAPTER 6

Weighting for ill health: the Nottingham Health Profile

Crispin Jenkinson

Introduction

The purpose of this chapter is two-fold. First, an outline will be made of methods by which items on health status measures may be weighted for severity. Secondly, the method in which one of the most frequently used generic health status questionnaires, the Nottingham Health Profile (NHP) (Hunt et al. 1986), was devised and the items weighted for severity will be described. It will be argued that the method of weighting the NHP is both complex and can lead to inaccuracies. The chapter will argue that simple weighting and scoring schemes may lose little in terms of accuracy over more complex systems and are essential if questionnaires of subjective health state are to become a part of routine evaluation.

Psychometric methods of scale construction

Questionnaires designed for use in the evaluation of subjective health state are typically constructed using methods developed within the field of psychology. The three most frequently employed psychometric weighting techniques are Likert scaling, Guttman scaling and Thurstone scaling. Traditionally, this had not been the case with many scales simply summing item scores, each of which has been given equal weight. This is the easiest solution to scale scoring, but overlooks the possibility that some items in the scale may be more important to the underlying construct than others in the scale (Bowling 1991). The decision by many researchers to adopt more complex forms of weighting for items was an attempt to gain greater precision in measurement.

A number of well utilized subjective health measures are based upon the principles of Likert scaling. The Arthritis Impact Measurement Scales 2 (AIMS2) (Meenan et al. 1992) and many of the scales on the Short-Form 36 Health Survey questionnaire (SF-36), are examples of Likert scaling (Ware & Sherbourne 1992). The SF-36 is reproduced in Chapter 7 of this text.

The construction of a Likert scale, which consists of a number of items, proceeds as follows: first, a pool of items is composed. These items may be produced through clinical or expert judgement, or through interviews with appropriate patient groups or lay people. The questionnaire constructed from this procedure is then administered to a sample of respondents. Each respondent is requested to not simply affirm or disaffirm the statements but to select from a number of responses to each item. Items may then be factor analyzed to determine whether they are all tapping a single underlying construct, or whether there are a number of underlying constructs being measured by the questionnaire. Factor analysis is a statistical technique that can be used to determine what items comprise a domain on a questionnaire, because they are tapping an underlying attribute. For example, a researcher may design a questionnaire to measure subjective health status, but on factor analysis may find the questionnaire has three factors. On inspection of the items the researcher may decide the questionnaire taps emotional problems, social problems and functional problems, and may decide to score these domains separately.

Once the areas measured by a questionnaire have been selected, researchers may wish to reduce the number of items in a scale to ensure both brevity and that items in a scale are the ones most strongly associated with the underlying attribute. This can be done by item-total score correlations, with items showing the highest correlation with the total score being retained in a questionnaire. Ideally this should be undertaken by correlating each question with the total of all the other items in the scale. Items which do not gain high correlations with the overall scale score should be removed as they may adversely influence the reliability of the scale. The internal reliability of the questionnaire can be assessed by a statistic known as Cronbach's alpha, which is an inter-item correlation statistic. The higher the alpha value the more confidence we may have that a questionnaire is tapping the proposed underlying construct. It is possible to use this statistic to reduce the number of items in a questionnaire. To do this the alpha statistic is calculated for the scale minus each item in turn. If removal of a certain item increases the value of alpha then the item may be dropped.

Guttman scaling is a scaling method in which degrees of attitude, disability or emotional state are ranked in order. This method of scaling has been used in the original Arthritis Impact Measurement Scales (Meenan 1982), the Index of Activities of Daily Living (Katz & Akpom 1976) and the Beck Depression Inventory (Beck et al. 1961). Guttman scaling begins with a large pool of items which are then reduced, on the basis of judgement by the researcher, to a relatively small sample of 10–20 items which are thought to span the range of the attitude or behaviour being assessed. It is crucial in Guttman scaling that items tap only a single underlying attribute, since the final score on a questionnaire designed using this method arises from the accumulated response to all items.

Streiner & Norman (1989) give the following as an example of Guttman scaling:

I am able to:

1. Walk across the room.
2. Climb the stairs.
3. Walk one block or more.
4. Walk more than a mile.

It is assumed in Guttman scaling that affirmation of, in the example above, item 4, would ensure the respondent would affirm 1–3. Similarly, affirmation of item 3 would ensure affirmation of items 1–2. It has been suggested that Guttman scaling is best suited to behaviours that are developmentally determined (e.g. crawling, standing, walking, running) where mastery of the lower order behaviours is necessary for mastery of the higher order ones (Streiner & Norman 1989). It may not, however, be ideally suited to the measurement of emotional wellbeing or impairments where loss of one function may not alter lower order functions, such as in stroke patients (Streiner & Norman 1989).

The developers of the Nottingham Health Profile (NHP) (Hunt et al. 1985, 1986) were critical of psychometric methods such as Likert and Guttman for use in developing subjective health indicators. They claimed that questionnaires produced by such methods were unduly complicated, and that more simple questionnaires, where items had simple dichotomous "yes/no" responses were more straightforward for respondents to understand, and complete.

The Nottingham Health Profile

In an attempt to develop a questionnaire that would be easy for respondents to complete the developers of the NHP used a similar technique to that of Bergner and colleagues in the development of the Sickness Impact Profile (SIP) (Bergner et al. 1981). Bergner and her colleagues had utilized Thurstone scaling in their attempt to develop a subjective health indicator. Hunt et al. (1986) argued

> There are a number of criticisms that can be made of existing measures . . . although not all of the following comments apply to each instrument. First, they are often long and complicated with ambiguous statements; second, scoring and weighting for seriousness often reflect the values of the physician not those of the lay person; thirdly, the focus of the measures may be on too narrow an area, for example disability; and fourthly, where the answers are summed to a single score or index this can be derived in many different ways and involve the addition of scores not logically related.

The Nottingham Health Profile was designed to overcome such problems.

The Nottingham Health Profile is a questionnaire consisting of two sections. The first section, containing 38 items, is intended to measure perceptions of ill health. The items are distributed between the areas of pain (8 items), physical mobility (8 items), emotional reactions (9 items), sleep disturbance (5 items), social isolation (5 items) and energy (3 items). Figure 6.1 gives examples of items on the NHP. The second section asks respondents to indicate whether or not their state of health affects activity in seven areas of everyday life: job or work, looking after the house, social life, home life, sex life, interests and hobbies, and holidays. Responses on part II are coded as a simple "yes/no", and no weighting is provided nor are any of the items summed together. Part II of the questionnaire has been used less extensively than part I.

The NHP has been utilized extensively. For example, it has been used in studies of the general population (Hunt et al. 1986, Brazier et al. 1992), on unemployed and re-employed men (McKenna & Payne 1989), on pregnant women (Hunt et al. 1986) and on patients with migraine (Jenkinson et al. 1988, Jenkinson & Fitzpatrick 1990), osteoarthritis (Hunt

Dimension	Item content (example)
Mobility	I have trouble getting up and down stairs and steps
Pain	I'm in pain when I'm sitting
Social isolation	I feel there is no one I am close to
Sleep	I lie awake for most of the night
Emotional reactions	I've forgotten what it is like to enjoy myself
Energy	I'm tired all the time

Figure 6.1 NHP domains and example item content.

et al. 1986), rheumatoid arthritis (Jenkinson & Fitzpatrick 1990, Fitzpatrick et al. 1991), peripheral vascular disease (Hunt et al. 1986) and in studies of cholecystectomy (Bardsley et al. 1992), heart/lung transplants (O'Brien et al. 1988) and clinical trials of anti-hypertensive medication (DeLame et al. 1989). A substantial number of projects that have included the NHP are summarized in Hunt et al. (1989). Data suggests that the measure is good at identifying people with chronic illnesses, and distinguishing between different conditions (Wilkin et al. 1992). Furthermore, recent work with the profile has suggested that the questionnaire can be scored in such a way as to gain a single index figure. This procedure requires the removal of certain items from the original 38 in the questionnaire. The revised scoring gives a "distress" score. The questionnaire can be administered in this new 24-item shortened format in order to gain a single index figure of health-related distress, which can be used in QALY type cost–utility analysis (McKenna et al. 1993).

One of the great advantages of questionnaires such as the NHP is the apparently low level of respondent burden. With the NHP this was achieved by adopting statements to which respondents answer either "yes" or "no". However, to provide greater measurement precision than could apparently be gained from simple summing of positive responses to items the designers decided to utilize weights. Each item carries a specific weight, ascribed to it by the originators from a weighting technique they refer to as Thurstone's method of paired comparisons (McKenna et al. 1981). This method of weighting is an operationalization of Thurstone's (1927) Law of Comparative Judgement, in which it is assumed that for each stimulus statement there exists a most frequently occurring response. "The basic assumption underlying the law of comparative judgement is that the degree to which any two stimuli can be discriminated is a direct function of the difference in their status as regards the attribute in question" (McIver & Carmines 1981). Thurstone is, thus, claiming that for any given set of statements there exists a *typical* response ordering, and, further, that the degree to which such statements can be differentiated is an indication of their proximity to the underlying attribute. Once the statements have been selected for the questionnaire, of course, it is possible for respondents to affirm all or none, or indeed any number, of the statements, as they all tap an underlying attribute (e.g. attitude to the church). However, it must be borne in mind that much of Thurstone's research was concerned with the measurement of psychological variables such as attitude (Thurstone 1928). It has been suggested that it is misleading to use Thurstone's method to attempt to scale statements that are, or could be viewed as, factual (Edwards 1957). The NHP contains factual statements (e.g. "I'm unable to walk at all") and it is suggested here that it is for this reason that the NHP contains illogical groups of (factual) statements. Thus, some of the statements contained in the mobility section of the NHP logically preclude subjects responding to other items. For example, an affirmation of the statement "I'm unable to walk at all" (with a weight value of 21.30) *technically* precludes positive responses to some other aspects of mobility. If a respondent affirms the statement that they are unable to walk, they should not, logically, be able to affirm the statements "I can only walk about indoors" (weight 11.54), and "I have trouble getting up and down stairs and steps" (weight 10.79), which make a total score of 22.33. Thus the score of a respondent with walking difficulties exceeds that of someone totally unable to walk.

Not only is Thurstone scaling essentially for use in attitude research, but it is advisable that statements chosen represent the entire spectrum of the affective scale of interest so that the items span the entire range of the attitudinal continuum under study. Further, items should not be included which are likely to be endorsed by almost everyone, or almost no-one (Edwards 1957). Both of these further assumptions are violated with the NHP. The originators themselves remark that the items "represent rather severe problems. This was found to be necessary in order to avoid picking up large numbers of false positives. However, it does mean that some milder forms of distress may not show up on the profile. Members of "normal" populations, or those with minor ailments may affirm very few statements" (Hunt et al. 1986). Indeed studies of the general population have shown the NHP to pick up only the most severe end of health-related problems (Kind & Carr-Hill 1987, Brazier et al. 1992).

Measurement problems in the NHP

So far, the weights given to the NHP have been criticized on theoretical grounds relating to the assumptions of Thurstone scaling. Due to the inappropriate use of Thurstone scaling there is a very small variance of values for each statement within every topic domain. This issue has been raised by Kind (1982). He argues that similar weights for different items should not be included in a measure as similar scores on different attitude statements would indicate a similar reflection to the attitudes, and hence this leads to tautological groups of statements.

Certainly the point that variance in weights is limited in the domains is easily verifiable. For example, there are only three statements for energy, with scale values of 39.2, 36.8 and 24.0. Likewise, the emotional reactions scale, which contains the largest number of items, has weight values ranging from 7.08 to 16.21, which is not a large variance. The variance of weights in Thurstone's work had a far greater spread, no doubt largely due to his intention to cover the gamut of attitudes to a particular phenomenon (e.g. Thurstone & Chave (1929) developed a scale to measure attitudes to the church. Item values covered a far greater spread than those in the NHP. Indeed values were as low as 0.2 and as high as 9.6. The proportional difference between these weights is substantially wider than those used for items on the NHP). As the statements in the NHP represent the severe end of health problems, and hence there is limited variance in weight values, it is really questionable as to whether there is any need for scaled weights.

The argument so far has suggested that there is little theoretical support for using Thurstone's method in order to gain weights for a questionnaire such as the NHP. Further, the claim that there is insufficient variance in the weights can be demonstrated empirically by a rescoring of the items on the NHP. This enables a comparison to be made between results gained by weighting against those gained simply by giving values of "0" and "1" to the responses of the questionnaire ("0" for a negative response, and "1" for a positive response).

Table 6.1 contains results gained from a study of the health status of patients presenting with migraine and rheumatoid arthritis (Jenkinson et al. 1988, Jenkinson 1991). Data on the NHP are provided in the form of weighting responses, as suggested by the designers of the NHP, and also by simply summing the number of affirmative answers in each dimension on the NHP and expressing this number as a percentage. The two

Table 6.1 NHP scores gained by summing item weights or summing dichotomous score expressed as a percentage (in parentheses) for migraine and rheumatoid arthritis patients.

	Migraine (n = 80)	RA (n = 68)
Mobility	3.84	55.38
	(4.38)	(61.38)
Pain	18.40	64.44
	(14.86)	(68.25)
Social isolation	15.87	26.78
	(15.60)	(25.00)
Sleep	30.51	51.42
	(30.20)	(53.80)
Emotional reactions	29.14	25.87
	(29.56)	(32.56)
Energy	41.64	63.00
	(42.33)	(63.67)

scores are therefore comparable as they both have a maximum score of 100.

Results gained from the two methods of scoring the questionnaire were correlated. No correlation was less than 0.98 (p < 0.0001) for any of the groups of respondents. Although a significant correlation between the two different methods of administration may be expected on any given domain, the very high strength of association found here would call into question the relevance of weighting items.

It has been suggested that although it may be appropriate to forego the use of weights in descriptive studies, it is imperative that the weights are used in studies in which change is being evaluated (Hunt & McKenna 1991). Sensitivity to change is an important aspect of health status measures and weights may be required to increase the "responsiveness" of measures such as the NHP. Data from a study of patients with rheumatoid arthritis who were followed up over time were analyzed to determine whether weighting substantially altered the results over simple dichotomous scoring. The Rheumatology Department of the Nuffield Orthopaedic Centre, Oxford, approached 102 consecutive patients diagnosed as having classic or definite rheumatoid arthritis and invited them to take part in a longitudinal study, of which the results reported here are based upon two interviews with each patient separated by a period of three months. Although no patient refused to take part at the first interview, one withdrew prior to the completion of the data-gathering phase of this study due to work commitments and one patient died during the course of the study. The final analysis, therefore, is based upon 100 respondents. Change scores were calculated using both the weighting procedure suggested by the NHP designers, and by simple scoring. The results are reported in Table 6.2.

Table 6.2 NHP mean change scores for rheumatoid arthritis patients, gained by summing item weights or dichotomous raw score expressed as a percentage (n = 100).

	Weighted change scores	Unweighted change scores
Mobility	1.32	1.86
Pain	2.61	2.48
Social isolation	−0.31	−0.20
Sleep	−3.87	−3.37
Emotional reactions	−1.38	−1.98
Energy	0.27	0.33

As can be seen, the extent of change indicated is similar for both procedures. Effect sizes were also calculated. This is recommended by Kazis et al. (1989) for providing an easily interpretable statistic to indicate the amount of change over time. Effect sizes were similar whether calculated using the weighted or unweighted values gained from the NHP. Furthermore, in this study data from the FLP were also analyzed, both with the data weighted and simply dichotomously scored. Again, similar results were gained for both of these methods (Jenkinson et al. 1991).

Discussion

The NHP has been extensively used. Work suggests that it can provide a valid and reliable picture of health state. However, the data presented here suggests that the complex weighting procedure adds little to the accuracy of the instrument, and may in fact detract from it. Although it is appropriate to assume that different health states reflect different degrees of seriousness, and hence should contribute differentially to overall scores, it must also be borne in mind that complex weighting systems make questionnaires unwieldy and unlikely candidates for routine use. Furthermore, many of the weighting techniques developed are designed for the evaluation of attitude, and may not be ideal candidates for the construction of health status profiles. Thurstone scaling is inappropriate for a questionnaire that contains statements which are non-attitudinal and which cover only the extreme end of the dimensions being measured. These are violations of the assumptions inherent in this method of weighting (Edwards 1957), and must cast at least some doubt on the validity of the weights on the questionnaire.

It has been argued here that the choice to scale items that are essentially factual with a method more appropriate for attitudes has meant that not only are weights insufficiently spread to be sensitive to health status differences, but logical inconsistencies exist within the NHP, whereby, for example, individuals who are unable to walk may score less than those who have difficulty walking. Further, another assumption of Thurstone scaling may be violated in the mobility category of the NHP, in that items should all reflect some underlying (unidimensional) construct. In the "physical mobility" category statements include difficulty with walking and dressing. It is suggested here that having difficulty dressing is a rather different problem from being unable to walk. One may not be able to walk because one is physically incapable of doing so, but may have difficulty dressing because of joint deformation in the hand, caused by RA. Kind (1982) similarly notes that items in the sleep category do not seem to tap a single underlying dimension. It is possible that weights in dimensions are similar because respondents, in the original weighting exercise for the NHP, regarded them to be of equal severity, but that they do not tap an underlying unidimensional construct. Thus, having difficulty walking about outside may be regarded as being as great a handicap as having difficulty dressing, but they may not co-exist on the hypothesized underlying unidimensional construct of "physical mobility". In the Sickness Impact Profile (Bergner et al. 1981) difficulty walking falls in the "ambulation" category, and difficulty dressing in the "bodycare" category.

Empirical evidence has been provided here that suggests that the weighting of items in the NHP by Thurstone's method is unsuccessful, as results remain remarkably similar whether responses are weighted or scored 1/0. Thus the weighting procedure adds very little, and may indeed be misleading. Similar findings have been reported for the Functional Limitations Profile (Jenkinson et al. 1991). Such findings provide support for the view that health measurement, in order to be useful, must also not be so complex as to make it unwieldy, or, indeed, untenable. The argument of this chapter is that simple scoring systems may be just as appropriate as complex methods of weighting. Furthermore, the decision of the designers of the NHP to limit the response set to a dichotomous "yes/no" format was in order to reduce respondent burden. However, despite the attempts of the developers to produce an instrument that was simple to understand and easy and quick to complete, other measures have achieved a higher response rate in community surveys. For example the SF-36 (see Chapter 7), which contains questions in a Likert type format, has gained higher completion rates than the NHP (Brazier et al. 1992). It has been suggested that far from the dichotomous response format being preferred by subjects, it can be viewed as difficult, if not impossible, to complete. Indeed, Donovan et al. (1993) have highlighted the difficulties many respondents have in completing the NHP, as the "yes/no" dichotomy can prevent people expressing their "true" feelings. Donovan and her colleagues found that although the restricted nature of the possible responses may lend itself to a potentially straightforward analysis, the results may be misleading as people have not been able to express how they really feel. From taped interviews, Donovan et al. found respondents often were unable to simply affirm or disaffirm statements on the questionnaire. For example, in response to the item "Things are getting me down", one respondent replied "I won't let them if I can. Can I put 'sometimes'?" Another respondent when asked to either affirm or not the statement "I have pain at night" replied "Not so much pain as discomfort, so what do I put?".

By adopting a complex scaling method, Hunt and her colleagues believed this meant that due weight would be given to the relative seriousness of items. The weight could be applied after the questions were asked by the researcher, and hence complex statements would not have to be posed nor complex judgements about health made by respondents. In practice, the statements lead people to think about their health, but then constrain their responses. On questionnaires utilizing Guttman and Likert type formats there is a greater choice of response.

Complex forms of weighting may provide an air of "scientific credibility" to health status measures, but they neither seem reliable nor appropriate for use in many circumstances where not only is a questionnaire needed that is easy to complete, but also easy to score. Simplicity in how questions are posed, and in the format of possible responses to items, is to be encouraged, but not to the extent that respondents can no longer answer questions in such a way as to reflect their perceived health state. For health status measures to be useful they must permit for ease of scoring and analysis, and be acceptable and meaningful to the demands of those completing them.

CHAPTER 7

The long and the short of it: the development of the SF-36 General Health Survey

Lucie Wright

Introduction

The purpose of this chapter is to provide a "natural history" of health status measures which have been developed from research undertaken initially by the RAND Corporation in the United States. In doing so the aim is to describe the genealogy of the short-form 36-item General Health Survey questionnaire (SF-36), one of the latest and most frequently used in the family of subjective health status measures. A copy of this questionnaire appears at the end of this chapter.

There has been a gradual shift away from a sole reliance upon clinical and laboratory measures of health and illness and a shift towards incorporating measurement of individuals' own assessment of their health. In the Health Insurance Experiment and the Medical Outcomes Study, the RAND Corporation endeavoured to develop instruments which could tap subjective assessment of functioning and wellbeing. One of the intentions of the research was to construct an instrument which could be administered to a wide range of illness groups, which took only a few minutes to complete, while at the same time fulfilling the psychometric requirements of validity and reliability.

The two RAND studies yielded a number of instruments, the longest of which was the Functioning and Well-being Profile and the shortest was the short-form 6 (SF-6). One of the earliest of the Medical Outcomes Study short-form general health survey instruments was the SF-20. This was a 20-item scale covering six health dimensions – physical functioning, rôle functioning, bodily pain, current health perceptions, social functioning and mental health. Although it satisfied the requirements of brevity and general applicability, its use in the field revealed a number of psycho-metric limitations. Addressing these led the Medical Outcomes Study research team to develop the SF-36 which, as the name suggests, involved a lengthening of the instrument from 20 to 36 items, thus almost doubling its length. In this chapter evidence relating to the psychometric and prac-tical properties of the SF-20 will be provided, including a discussion of the instrument's limitations which led to its replacement by the SF-36. The psychometric and practical properties of the 36-item scale are then dis-cussed, and its advantages and limitations outlined.

The health insurance experiment and the Medical Outcomes Study long-form instruments

General health surveys utilized in the Health Insurance Experiment and in the Medical Outcomes Study were the precursors of the short-form instruments. The distinctive feature of both studies was the decision to collect patient-assessed outcome measures as well as traditional clinical and laboratory measures of health and illness.

The RAND Health Insurance Experiment (HIE) was a US federal govern-ment funded study which ran between 1974 and 1982 to examine the effect of health payment systems on the use of health services. Approxi-mately 4,000 people aged 14 to 61, representative of the general popula-tion of the area where they lived (Brook et al. 1983), were enrolled into the study from six sites. Participants were followed for three years, 30 per cent of whom were followed up for a further two years. One of the major findings of the study was that those enrolled in a co-payment scheme made a third fewer medical visits and were hospitalized a third less often than those receiving care free at the point of entry. To deter-mine whether those receiving "free" care were healthier as a result, measures were developed to evaluate the effect of cost-sharing on health status (Brook et al. 1983). These measures included instruments to assess subjective health. The HIE health questionnaire contained 108 items which were administered at entry and on leaving the study. Self-assessed general health was measured on five dimensions: physical functioning, rôle functioning, mental health, social contacts, and health perceptions. Results led to two main conclusions: that free care did not improve health status regardless of how it was measured (Brook et al. 1983); and that "the HIE clearly demonstrated the potential of scales constructed from self-administered surveys as reliable and valid tools for assessing changes in health status for both adults and children in the general population" (Ware 1992: 5). The HIE health questionnaire consequently provided the background for the Medical Outcomes Study patient-assessed health measures.

The Medical Outcomes Study (MOS) was a two year prospective study with two major aims. First, to determine whether variations in patient outcomes could be explained by variations in system of care, clinician specialty, and clinicians' technical and interpersonal style. A second purpose of the study was to develop instruments for the routine monitoring of patient outcomes in medical practice, specifically, self-administered questionnaires and generic scales (Tarlov et al. 1989). Random samples of physicians were drawn from different health care settings in Boston, Massachusetts; Chicago, Illinois and Los Angeles, California. Over 22,000 patients who consulted the sampled doctors during nine day screening periods between February and November 1986 completed a screening form in which they evaluated their health status and treatment. Of these, over 3,000 patients with one or more of a number of specific health problems or "tracer" conditions, including diabetes mellitus, hypertension, heart disease, and depression, were selected for the longitudinal study (McHorney et al. in press). Over the following two years hospitalizations and treatments were monitored and the health status of these patients was repeatedly measured. The study was then able to correlate the structures (e.g. the method of payment), the processes (e.g. the clinician's interpersonal style) and the outcomes (both clinical/laboratory measures and patient-assessed) of medical treatment.

The largest set of MOS health measures included in a single questionnaire, the Functioning and Well-Being Profile (MOSFWBP), was administered in the baseline Patient Assessment Questionnaire (PAQ) (Stewart et al. 1992a) to patients who were identified as having one or more tracer conditions. These patients were asked to complete the profile at the start of the longitudinal phase of the study. This measure is recommended for studies in which the "full set" of MOS scales is required (Stewart et al. 1992d). It includes 35 scales and 149 items measuring physical and rôle functioning, social, family and sexual functioning, mobility, psychological distress/wellbeing, cognitive functioning, health perceptions, health distress, energy/fatigue, sleep, pain, and physical/psycho-physiological symptoms (Stewart et al. 1992d). Due to the length and breadth of this profile, completion takes an estimated 30 to 37 minutes. The full PAQ, including the MOSFWB Profile, amounts to 245 items.

Medical Outcomes Study short-form instruments

The Short-Form General Health Survey (SF-20) was developed within the MOS in the quest for a generic health status measure which could satisfy a number of potentially conflicting criteria. Ideally the authors wished to develop a measure which was short enough to be completed quickly yet was also comprehensive (covering as many dimensions of health as possible) with psychometrically sound, multi-item scales (Stewart et al. 1988). Part of the rationale behind the pursuit of short-form health status measures was the idea of "outcomes management" whereby clinical, financial and health outcomes data could form a national database with which to inform decision-making (Ellwood, 1988). In this schema patient-generated outcomes data is then elicited from short-form subjective health status instruments. Within the MOS the aim was to develop and refine the SF-20 as a method for assessing functional status and wellbeing while at the same time examining its sensitivity, as a generic measure, to the impact of disease and treatments (Tarlov et al. 1989).

Development of the SF-20 General Health Survey questionnaire

The HIE provided the basis for the 20-item short-form instrument. Eighteen items were drawn from the parent instrument. The remaining items were single item measures of social functioning and bodily pain that were developed following experience with the similar measures in the HIE (Stewart et al. 1988). Like any health status measure, the SF-20 is required to fulfil a number of criteria if it is to be useful. A measure should be:
   - appropriate for the research issue in terms of the content and dimensions of health covered and in terms of the levels of health or ill health it covers;
   - reliable;
   - valid;
   - practically useful (Bergner & Rothman 1987: 194);
   - sensitive to change.

An examination of the extent to which the SF-20 fulfils the above criteria helps to highlight the shortcomings of the instrument and hence the decision to supersede it with the SF-36.

One of the aims of the MOS was to develop a measure which would be appropriate to general population groups as well as to patient groups (Stewart & Ware 1992). The MOS instruments are described as "generic", in that they are intended to assess health concepts that represent basic human values that are relevant to everyone's health status and wellbeing regardless of age, disease or treatment group (Ware 1992, Ware 1987). The SF-20 has been used in a variety of general population and patient groups. Of the core 18 items drawn from the HIE questionnaire, 17 were included in a telephone interview study. This was conducted by Louis Harris Associates in 1984 and involved 2000 adults in US households, half of whom were enrolled in Health Maintenance Organisations (HMOs) and half in Fee for Service (FFS) systems. The results provided a general population sample with which patient samples from the MOS could be compared. In the Medical Outcomes Study all 20 items of the instrument were administered to a randomly selected half of the total screening sample totalling approximately 11,000 adults (Stewart & Ware 1992). Results are reported elsewhere in relation to chronic medical conditions (Stewart et al. 1989) and to depression (Wells et al. 1989). Other studies have also utilized the SF-20 and contributed to assessment of its validity and reliability (Bindman et al. 1990). Clearly an instrument such as the SF-20 can only be considered appropriate for a wide range of population and patient groups if it is adequate to detect such a wide range of health status groups (Bergner & Rothman 1987).

Assessing the reliability of an instrument entails determination of the extent to which measurements of individuals obtained under different circumstances (on different occasions, by different observers, or by similar tests) yield similar results. Reliability is often described as a measure of the proportion of the variability in scores which was due to true differences between individuals (Streiner & Norman 1989), as opposed to differences due to random error. As McHorney and colleagues point out with regard to reliability testing, it is how a measure performs in a particular sample or application which is more important than its general performance (McHorney et al. in press). The internal consistency of the SF-20 has been examined in a variety of patient group samples. Internal consistency indicates the homogeneity of the items of a scale and is measured by the degree to which they correlate with each other and with the overall score (Streiner & Norman 1989). On the SF-20 two health dimensions, bodily pain and social functioning, are measured by single items which clearly prohibit this type of reliability measurement. On the other four multi-item scales reliability coefficients ranged from 0.76 upwards. This was lower, but not much lower, than those gained for the full-length long-form parent profiles (Stewart et al. 1988). Reliabilities at this level satisfy the minimum requirements for group assessment.

Test-retest reliability of the SF-20 was evaluated in a study in which there was a four month period between the two measurements (Stewart et al. 1992a). However, data from this study have not yet been reported and, given the time lapse between administrations, is unlikely to contribute to the evidence supporting the reliability of the measure. Given the vast amount of data collected it is unfortunate that test-retest reliability could not have been investigated or reported.

Evidence of validity is required in order to ascertain whether a test is measuring what is intended (Streiner & Norman 1989). Streiner & Norman state that "validating a scale is really a process whereby we determine the degree of confidence we can place on inferences we make about people based on their scores from that scale" (Streiner & Norman 1989: 108). Three broad types of validity testing – (a) content, (b) criterion, and (c) construct – are usually described, each addressing this same issue of confidence.

(a) The content validity of a scale may be assessed by answering the question – are all aspects of a definition of a concept represented? Ware has provided a set of minimum standards by which to evaluate health measures (Ware 1987). The full-length long-form MOSFWB Profile is composed of 12 health dimensions. The existing literature was used as the definitional standard against which to compare these health concepts (Stewart et al. 1992b).

Stewart and colleagues note the complexity of health research concepts and the definitional problems this imposes. This, they argue, means that single item measures are unlikely to be adequate to operationalize a construct (Stewart et al. 1992a). It is perhaps surprising, therefore, that of the six health dimensions in the SF-20 two are measured by single item scales: social functioning and bodily pain. As Ware and colleagues point out there is often a trade-off between depth and breadth when developing measurement instruments (Ware et al. 1992b), that is, between the precision with which a health concept is measured and its comprehensiveness and content validity. Using single item measures is one way of limiting length without compromising the breadth of the instrument. The SF-6, a six item questionnaire, was developed to consider and examine this issue. Although it is a broad measure in that it includes six dimensions of health: physical, social and rôle functioning, bodily pain, mental health, or more precisely psychological distress, and general health perceptions, its depth is limited to the precision achievable using a single item for each concept (Ware et al. 1992a). When compared to six long-form multi-item MOS scales the SF-6 was found to be, as expected, less reliable and less able to detect small differences between groups. Furthermore it was less sensitive to change over time in individual patients (Ware et al. 1992a). The source of several of the problems associated with the SF-20 was the inclusion of single item measures for two of the health dimensions. Accordingly one of the goals of the SF-36 was to enhance content validity (Ware & Sherbourne 1992) by expanding all dimensions into multi-item scales.

(b) The criterion validity of a scale refers to the extent to which a measure correlates with a "gold standard" measure of that concept. That is, the extent to which an instrument fares favourably when compared to a tried, tested and accepted alternative measure of the same concepts. For the SF-20 this was done by comparing scales to the long-form versions of the scales (Stewart et al. 1992b). Although results do not appear to be readily available, it would be reasonable to expect that they would reveal that scales derived from longer instruments were highly correlated with those same long form instruments.

(c) Construct validity refers to the extent to which measures correlate with measures of other variables in hypothesized ways. The MOS examined the differences in scores associated with the presence of a variety of chronic medical conditions (Stewart et al. 1989) and depression (Wells et al. 1989) in order to test the hypotheses about the relative effects of those conditions (Stewart et al. 1992b). Results provided evidence for the construct validity of the SF-20, for example, as expected physical functioning scores were higher, indicating better health on this domain, for hypertensive patients than for those with myocardial infarction or heart failure (Stewart et al. 1989).

Two practical considerations when using health status measures are the respondent burden involved and the mode of administration (Bergner & Rothman 1987). Part of the rationale behind the development of short-form measures was a reduction in respondent burden, from the 30 minutes plus taken to complete the HIE health scale or the Sickness Impact Profile (Bergner et al. 1981) to a length which would be of practical use in the clinic setting (Stewart et al. 1988: 724). To this extent the SF-20 was a success; respondent burden was reduced by about 80 per cent (Stewart et al. 1988). Another aim in the development of short-form measures was flexibility in mode of administration. The SF-20 is able to be administered largely by self completion with little need for face-to-face or telephone interview (Ware 1992).

To be able to detect change in scores, scales must be sensitive to both improvement or deterioration in health status (Kazis et al. 1989). A floor effect was found with the SF-20, particularly on single item dimensions in a study of severely ill patients (Bindman et al. 1990). A group of very ill patients completed the SF-20 at baseline and six months later. At the second administration of the SF-20 patients were also asked transition questions; i.e. they were asked to directly assess how their health had changed on the six dimensions of the short-form measure. Over 11 per cent of patients were at the floor recording the lowest possible score (i.e. the worst health) on one or more dimensions of the SF-20 at baseline, and six months later reported that their health had become worse. There was no scope on the SF-20 for recording this deterioration in health. This problem was particularly found for those dimensions measured by single item scales. A number of patients who recorded zero for pain or social functioning reported a deterioration in these dimensions of their health as measured on the corresponding transition questions. As well as low baseline scores on the SF-20 prohibiting the recognition of larger declines in function, Bindman and colleagues found that low baseline scores were associated with smaller falls in follow-up scores. Even more a cause for concern, however, was the discovery that when patients' baseline scores on a dimension were at or near zero, the change in scores became positive despite a reported deterioration in health on the respective dimension (Bindman et al. 1990). The authors conclude from this work that while severely ill patients are willing to complete the SF-20, the instrument may not be sufficiently responsive to changes in their health status (Bindman et al. 1990). The floor effect problem may not be so important when administered to more healthy populations, although a ceiling effect may prohibit the recognition of improvements in health.

In summary, while the SF-20 satisfied the search for a short, easily administered, generic health status measure a number of limitations became apparent in use. Most significantly the inclusion of single item scales for bodily pain and social functioning made these domains insensitive to different health states and changes over time. The presence of a significant floor effect among severely ill patients created an instrument bias against recording a decline in health in the very group of patients among whom a detection of deterioration in health may be most important.

Development of the SF-36 General Health Survey questionnaire

It was the problems with the SF-20 which led to the development of the SF-36 and precipitated a return to longer measures. In a recent paper, MOS researchers stated that "The MOS 36-item Short-Form Health Survey (SF-36) was constructed to broaden the health concepts measured and improve measurement precision for each concept over that achieved by the SF-20" (McHorney et al. 1993). This section will discuss the extent to which the SF-36 has been able to do so and the degree to which it achieves the ideal criteria for a useful health status measure. That is, the extent to which it fulfils the requirements of validity, reliability, appropriateness, practicality, and sensitivity to change. In doing so attention will be drawn to the limitations associated with its precursor, the SF-20, and its success in addressing these problems, in particular those associated with single item scales and floor effects.

Validity testing has been carried out in the US and in the UK and has included examination of the (a) content, (b) criterion and (c) construct validity of the instrument.

(a) One of the aims of the SF-36 was to improve the content validity of the short-form measures compared to the 20-item scale. To achieve this the number of dimensions of health was increased to eight and the number of items almost doubled to 36 (see Table 7.1). In terms of the validity of the scales it is worth briefly describing how each was developed and modified from the SF-20 version.

The two single item scales, bodily pain and social functioning, were developed into multi-item versions.

– *Bodily pain:* the SF-20 asked about the intensity of bodily pain, whereas the SF-36 also asks about the degree to which pain interferes with normal functional abilities (Sherbourne 1992b). These two items were drawn from the 12-item pain battery in the MOSFWB

Table 7.1 Health concepts and number of questionnaire items per concept, MOS short–form health surveys.

	Number of items	
	SF–20	SF–36
Health concepts		
Functional status		
Physical functioning	6	10
Social functioning	1	2
Role functioning	2	
Physical		4
Mental		3
Wellbeing		
Mental health	5	5
Energy / fatigue	–	4
Pain	1	2
Overall evaluation of health		
General health perceptions	5	5
Change in health		
Change in health	–	1
Total	20	36

Profile which in turn was adapted from the Wisconsin Brief Pain Questionnaire (Daut et al. 1983) and the Health Information Study Questionnaire.

– *Social functioning:* the social functioning dimension was expanded to a two item scale in the SF-36 tapping two types of health-related effects on social functioning: first, the extent to which physical or emotional health problems limit interaction with others, and secondly, the changes in usual levels of social activity due to changes in health (Sherbourne 1992a). The MOS developed their own set of four questions on social functioning for the MOSFWB profile, two of which were utilized in the SF-36.

Multi-item scales in the SF-20 were also modified for the SF-36.

– *Physical functioning:* the physical functioning scale used in the SF-20 was composed of six items covering seven levels of physical functioning. For the SF-36 the measure was increased to the full long-form ten item scale covering 21 levels, making detection of small differences in function possible (Ware & Sherbourne 1992). Items were adapted from "nine existing measures of physical functioning" (Stewart & Kamberg 1992: 90). The MOSFWB Profile is composed of three physical functioning measures: a ten item physical functioning scale, a single item satisfaction with physical ability measure, and a two item mobility measure. Although the authors recommend using all three measures together (Stewart & Kamberg 1992), the SF-36 contains only the ten item scale.

– *Mental health:* the basis for the MOSFWB Profile was the Mental Health Inventory developed for the HIE and was composed of 38 items (Stewart et al. 1992e). A five item version was constructed from those questions in the Mental Health Inventory which best predicted the summary score for the 38-item set (Ware & Sherbourne 1992). This shortened version was utilized in the SF-20 and was retained unchanged in the SF-36.

– *Rôle functioning:* for the SF-20 a two item scale was taken from the HIE rôle functioning scale. As this proved to be a rather coarse scale (Ware & Sherbourne 1992) a number of changes were made for the SF-36. The rôle functioning dimension was expanded into two in order to capture rôle limitations due to physical health (four items) and emotional health (three items). New scales were created following a pilot study using items from published questionnaires and additional open-ended questions (Sherbourne et al. 1992).

– *Vitality:* a four item scale of vitality (energy level and fatigue) was added to the SF-36, a dimension of health not included in the SF-20. As with the mental health dimension, items were drawn from the Mental Health Inventory fielded in the HIE (Ware & Sherbourne 1992).

– *General health perceptions:* the five item current health sub-scale of the 26-item Health Perceptions Questionnaire (HPQ) utilized in the HIE was also used for the SF-20. It was decided to use a more comprehensive sample of items from the HPQ for the SF-36. Instead five items from the General Health Rating Index (GHRI), itself developed from the HPQ, were used (Stewart et al. 1992c, Ware & Sherbourne 1992).

– *Change in health:* a single item measuring change in health in the previous year was also included in the SF-36, although this item is not used to score any of the health dimensions (Ware & Sherbourne 1992).

(b) In the absence of criteria for the construction and validation of health scales such as the SF-36, the criterion for each scale was the full length MOS parent version (Ware & Sherbourne 1992). Criterion validity of the SF-36 has been examined on the Oxford Healthy Life Survey (Wright et al. 1992) data in which the general health perceptions item, asking people to define their health in general from "excellent" through to "poor", was used as the criterion against which the other items were tested. Although it is not common practice to use an item from a questionnaire to evaluate the criterion validity of that measure, the item is one which has been used in other studies to evaluate the validity of other instruments (Hunt et al. 1981, Doll et al. 1993) and, moreover, the item contributes to only one dimension and therefore does not contribute to the scale scores for the other seven dimensions. Results from this analysis provide evidence for the criterion validity of the instrument on a general population sample (Jenkinson et al. 1994). See Figures 7.1. and 7.2.

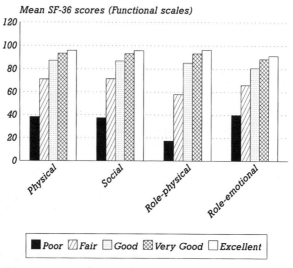

Figure 7.1 SF-36 functional scales broken down by overall perceived health.

(c) Construct validity of the SF-36 has been measured by comparing scores with hypothesized score distributions. As expected, men, higher social classes, younger age groups, those without chronic illness and those who had not consulted their general practitioner

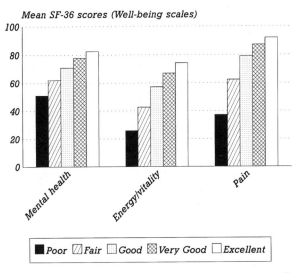

Figure 7.2 SF-36 wellbeing scales broken down by overall perceived health.

within the last two weeks scored higher than others, indicating better health (Brazier et al. 1992, Jenkinson et al. 1993a, 1993b). In order to assess convergent and discriminant validity Brazier and colleagues compared the SF-36 with the Nottingham Health Profile. Comparable dimensions of the two instruments generally correlated well (with the exception of the items measuring social functioning/ isolation, which were each addressing different aspects of social wellbeing) while item to own scale correlation was higher than item to other scale correlation (Brazier et al. 1992). In the United States, the SF-36 has undergone validity testing within the MOS using both psychometric and clinical criteria. Psychometric criteria were used to assess the extent to which each of the eight dimensions were indicators of the two major, underlying concepts of physical health and mental health (McHorney et al. 1993). This was done by measuring the validity of each scale and comparing it to the "most valid scale" for that dimension, that is, the scale which shared the most variance with either the physical or mental component of health (McHorney et al. 1993: 253). By doing so it was possible to estimate the degree to which a scale was a valid measure of physical and/or mental health status. Validity was also measured using clinical criteria; in order to investigate hypothesized relationships between patients, the SF-36 was administered to four patient groups each differing in physical and/or mental health status. It was expected that scales measuring physical health (i.e. physical functioning, rôle limitations due to physical health and bodily pain) would be most valid in distinguishing between groups differing in severity of chronic medical conditions, while scales measuring general mental health (i.e. the mental health scale and rôle limitations due to emotional problems) would be most valid in distinguishing between groups differing in the presence and severity of psychiatric disorders. Results indicated that both psychometric and clinical tests provided consistent information about the underlying nature of each scale and the degree to which each scale measured that component (McHorney et al. 1993). The SF-36, like the SF-20, is intended for use with both general population and patient groups. It has been used in two general population studies in the UK, in Sheffield (Brazier et al. 1992), and in Oxford (Jenkinson et al. 1993a, 1993b), both using lists of patients registered with a general practitioner as sampling frames. In addition, it has been used in patient groups in the UK and the US (McHorney et al. in press, Garrett et al. 1993a, 1993b). Again, as with the SF-20, each health dimension is given equal weight although it has been pointed out that the rationale for this was not based on patients' views as to the relative importance of each (Williams 1992).

The internal reliability of items on the SF-36 has been tested in a number of applications and reported both in the US and the UK. In the latter, internal reliability estimates have been calculated for general population groups, items within dimensions have been found to be highly correlated (Brazier et al. 1992, Jenkinson et al. 1993a). Alpha coefficients, an indicator of inter-item correlation, ranged from 0.73 (for social functioning) to 0.96 (for rôle limitation, physical and emotional, and vitality) in the Sheffield study, and from 0.76 (for social functioning) to 0.90 (for physical functioning) in the Oxford study. Using the MOS data, internal reliability has been examined across a range of sociodemographic groups and among patients of varying disease severity. The range of reliability coefficients was between 0.65 (for the general health scale) among the patient group with psychiatric and complicated medical disease, and 0.94 (for the physical functioning scale) among a number of patient groups (McHorney et al. in press). A Cronbach's alpha coefficient of 0.65 falls below the recommended 0.70 for the purposes of comparing groups (Nunnally 1978). This suggests that there may be reliability problems when the SF-36 is utilized among those with clinical complications or who are very ill.

There is less published data available on the reliability of the SF-36 over different time periods compared to results on its internal reliability. It has been argued that test-retesting of patient groups is problematic as it is difficult to assess whether score changes are due to measurement error or due to true improvement/deterioration in the health of the group (Ruta et al. 1993). This form of reliability has been assessed in a general population; Brazier and colleagues analyzed test-retest reliability at two weeks and found scores were highly correlated, with mean differences not clinically significant (Brazier et al. 1992). Test-retest studies from the MOS have yet to be published.

The number of items on the SF-36 is almost double that on the SF-20. This has practical implications. However, although respondent burden is increased this does not appear to have adversely affected response rates to those surveys which have included the instrument (Brazier et al. 1992, Wright et al. 1992), nor the proportion of missing values for each item (Brazier et al. 1992). It should be noted that higher rates of missing data have been reported for some social groups such as the elderly (Brazier et al. 1992, McHorney et al. in press), those with less than nine years of education, black patients, and those in poverty (McHorney et al. in press). As with the SF-20 the 36-item questionnaire was designed for self-administration, by telephone, or by interview (Ware & Sherbourne 1992).

By comparing clinically severe groups, results from construct validity tests also provided guidelines for interpreting score differences in each scale. However, as the authors themselves point out, the extent to which this is practical and meaningful is limited as differences are so large as to potentially render them meaningless (McHorney et al. 1993). One of the main reasons for the development of the SF-36 was the issue of ceiling and, more especially, floor effects. The degree to which these effects have been addressed by the SF-36 has been examined in the US where floor effects were observed only for the two rôle functioning scales, the most coarse of the scales, and were highest among the sickest patients (McHorney et al. 1993a). Ceiling effects were also most substantial for the two rôle functioning scales as the absence of rôle limitations is the highest level of the rôle functioning scales. There was also a substantial ceiling effect for the social functioning scale (McHorney et al. in press).

In summary, according to researchers on the MOS, efforts to increase the precision of the SF-36 by increasing the range of health measured for most concepts compared to the SF-20 were largely successful (McHorney in press). Evidence for the validity and reliability of the SF-36 is certainly accumulating both here in the UK and in the US. However, there remains much to be learned about the instrument's use in measuring subjective health status in a variety of settings and patient groups.

Conclusions

An enormous amount of time and energy and vast quantities of money have gone into the development of the MOS short-form instruments. The most recent and widely utilized measure, the SF-36 health survey questionnaire, is being used in a wide variety of circumstances and with increasing frequency in the UK and the US and is currently being translated into a number of languages for use across the world (Aaronson et al. 1992). It appears to be acceptable to patient and general population groups as response rates have been high in surveys that have included the instrument. It covers a wide range of areas that may be affected by ill health and has been found to be more sensitive to lower levels of disability than the Nottingham Health Profile (Brazier et al. 1992). Tests of validity and reliability to date look promising, although relatively little work has been carried out on the instrument's sensitivity to changes in health either in patient or population groups. However, not all is rosy. While many of the problems associated with the SF-20 have been addressed, some problems remain. Little is as yet known about how meaningful variations in scores are; to date only huge score differences have been proffered (McHorney et al. 1993) and smaller score differences remain open to interpretation. However, the availability of normative data, gathered from well-defined and representative samples of the population of interest, has made comparison and interpretation of scale scores possible (Ware et al. 1993). In terms of reliability, only one health dimension of the SF-36, physical functioning, consistently met minimum standards for use on an individual patient level (McHorney et al. in press); this has implications for its suitability in routine individual patient assessment in clinical practice. Issues pertaining to the validity of the instrument persist.

CONCLUSIONS

There are health-related areas that are not encompassed by the dimensions of the questionnaire. Sleep, for example, is an aspect of health which can be highly sensitive to both physical and mental wellbeing, and, conversely, can be indicative of health status. However, although items referring to sleep are included in the long-form MOSFWB Profile, it was omitted from the short-form versions. Other dimensions in the long-form measure excluded from the short-form scales include family and sexual functioning, and physical and psycho-physiological symptoms (Stewart et al. 1992d). In order to address the floor effect found in the SF-20, Bindman and colleagues recommend that the number of questions used to evaluate each dimension be increased (Bindman et al. 1990). This was the strategy adopted by the MOS researchers. However, the substantial floor effects detected on the two rôle functioning scales (McHorney et al. in press) of the SF-36 suggest that there is still some way to go before an instrument is developed which can be used to detect changes in health status in individuals and groups who range from physically and psychologically "healthy", through to those with complicated physical and mental illness. A number of modifications to the SF-36 have been suggested. These would increase the length of the instrument and hence respondent burden, and could involve the use of "supplemental batteries" of items for specific patient groups such as the severely ill (McHorney et al. in press). There remains scope for the further development of health status measurement scales, both within the MOS and elsewhere. However the short-form scales have come a long way since the Health Insurance Experiment and evidence of the validity and reliability of the SF-36 continues to accumulate.

The Short Form 36 Health Survey Questionnaire (SF-36)

The following questions ask for your views about your health, how you feel and how well you are able to do your usual activities. If you are unsure about how to answer any questions, please give the best answer you can and make any of your own comments if you like.

(Please tick one)

1. In general, would you say your health is:

    Excellent ☐
    Very good ☐
    Good ☐
    Fair ☐
    Poor ☐

2. **Compared to one year ago,** how would you rate your health in general **now**?

    Much better now than one year ago ☐
    Somewhat better now than one year ago ☐
    About the same ☐
    Somewhat worse now than one year ago ☐
    Much worse now than one year ago ☐

3. HEALTH AND DAILY ACTIVITIES

The following questions are about activities you might do during a typical day.
Does your health limit you in these activities? If so, how much?

(Please tick one box on each line)

		Yes, limited a lot	Yes, limited a little	No, not limited at all
a)	**Vigorous activities**, such as running, lifting heavy objects, participating in strenuous sports	☐	☐	☐
b)	**Moderate activities**, such as moving a table, pushing a vacuum cleaner, bowling or playing golf	☐	☐	☐
c)	Lifting or carrying groceries	☐	☐	☐
d)	Climbing **several** flights of stairs	☐	☐	☐
e)	Climbing **one** flight of stairs	☐	☐	☐
f)	Bending, kneeling or stooping	☐	☐	☐
g)	Walking **more than a mile**	☐	☐	☐
h)	Walking **half a mile**	☐	☐	☐
i)	Walking **100 yards**	☐	☐	☐
j)	Bathing and dressing yourself	☐	☐	☐

4. During the **past 4 weeks,** have you had any of the following problems with your work or other regular daily activities **as a result of your physical health**?

(Answer Yes or No to each question)

		Yes	No
a)	Cut down on the **amount of time** you spent on work or other activities	☐	☐
b)	**Accomplished less** than you would like	☐	☐
c)	Were limited in the **kind** of work or other activities	☐	☐
d)	Had **difficulty** performing the work or other activities (eg. it took extra effort)	☐	☐

107

5. During the **past 4 weeks**, have you had any of the following problems with your work or other regular daily activities **as a result of any emotional problems** (such as feeling depressed or anxious)?

(Answer Yes or No to each question)

		Yes	No
a)	Cut down on the **amount of time** you spent on work or other activities	☐	☐
b)	**Accomplished less** than you would like	☐	☐
c)	Didn't do work or other activities as **carefully** as usual	☐	☐

(Please tick one)

6. During the **past 4 weeks**, to what extent has your physical health or emotional problems interfered with your normal social activities with family, friends, neighbours or groups?

Not at all	☐
Slightly	☐
Moderately	☐
Quite a bit	☐
Extremely	☐

7. How much **bodily** pain have you had during the **past 4 weeks**?

None	☐
Very mild	☐
Mild	☐
Moderate	☐
Severe	☐
Very severe	☐

8. During the **past 4 weeks**, how much did **pain** interfere with your normal work (including work both outside the home and housework)?

Not at all	☐
A little bit	☐
Moderately	☐
Quite a bit	☐
Extremely	☐

These questions are about how you feel and how things have been with you **during the past month**. (For each question, please indicate the one answer that comes closest to the way you have been feeling).

(Please tick one box on each line)

9. How much time during **the past month**:

		All of the time	Most of the time	A good bit of the time	Some of the time	A little of the time	None of the time
a)	Did you feel full of life?	☐	☐	☐	☐	☐	☐
b)	Have you been a very nervous person?	☐	☐	☐	☐	☐	☐
c)	Have you felt so down in the dumps that nothing could cheer you up?	☐	☐	☐	☐	☐	☐
d)	Have you felt calm and peaceful?	☐	☐	☐	☐	☐	☐
e)	Did you have a lot of energy?	☐	☐	☐	☐	☐	☐
f)	Have you felt downhearted and low?	☐	☐	☐	☐	☐	☐
g)	Did you feel worn out?	☐	☐	☐	☐	☐	☐
h)	Have you been a happy person?	☐	☐	☐	☐	☐	☐
i)	Did you feel tired?	☐	☐	☐	☐	☐	☐
j)	Has your **health limited your social activities** (like visiting friends or close relatives)?	☐	☐	☐	☐	☐	☐

10. Please choose the answer that best describes how **true** or **false** each of the following statements is for you.

(Please tick one box on each line)

		Definitely true	Mostly true	Not sure	Mostly false	Definitely false
a)	I seem to get ill more easily than other people	☐	☐	☐	☐	☐
b)	I am as healthy as anybody I know	☐	☐	☐	☐	☐
c)	I expect my health to get worse	☐	☐	☐	☐	☐
d)	My health is excellent	☐	☐	☐	☐	☐

Reproduced by kind permission of the Health Outcomes Institute, Minneapolis, USA.

CHAPTER 8

Measuring functional limitations and sickness impact: a critical review of the FLP and SIP

Simon J. Williams

Introduction

Recent years have witnessed a growing interest in the measurement of health status and the evaluation of health care. Indeed, a proliferation of instruments now exists spanning functional disability, psychological wellbeing, social health, quality of life and life satisfaction, pain measurement and general health measurement (McDowell & Newell 1987, Bowling 1991). One of the most well known and extensively evaluated health status instruments to date, however, is the Sickness Impact Profile (SIP) (Bergner et al. 1981). Indeed, as McDowell & Newell (1987) comment, this scale is something of a gold standard against which other measures are judged.

Hence, this chapter discusses the development, nature and testing of the SIP and its UK equivalent the Functional Limitations Profile (FLP). In addition, it also discusses its application in a variety of research contexts and across different patient groups. Finally, it discusses some of the limitations, as well as the strengths, of this instrument and provides some cautionary remarks on its use in research and assessment. A copy of the FLP appears at the end of this chapter.

The SIP and FLP: nature, development and testing

The SIP was developed as a measure of perceived health status for use as an outcome measure for health care evaluation across differing types and severities of illness, and across socio-demographic and cultural sub-groups (Bergner et al. 1981). It was designed to be sensitive enough to detect changes or differences in health status that occur over time or between groups and was intended for use in measuring outcomes of health care in health surveys, in programme planning and policy formulation, and in monitoring patient progress.

The SIP measures sickness in relation to its impact upon behaviour (i.e. sickness-related dysfunction), rather than disease or subjective perceptions of illness. Its concentration upon behaviour is claimed to hold several advantages over feelings and clinical reports. First, feeling states are variable, hard to measure and are not amenable to external validation due to their subjectivity. Secondly, clinical assessments are either limited to patients under care, or else require medical interpretations of respondent-reported symptoms. In contrast, behavioural reports can be verified by observation and can be obtained whether or not a patient is receiving care. In addition, they may also be less subject to cultural bias than reports of feeling states (Bergner et al. 1976, McDowell & Newell 1987).

The items included in the SIP all focus upon changes in performance rather than capacity. In other words, they are concerned with what a person does or does not do, rather than with what they can or cannot do. The behaviours included in the profile are claimed to represent "universal patterns" of limitations that may be affected by disease or sickness, irrespective of the specific conditions, treatments, individual characteristics or prognoses concerned (Bergner et al. 1976, McDowell & Newell 1987).

Initial work on the SIP began in 1972. The instrument was developed on the basis of a literature review, statements collected from health professionals and interviews with healthy and ill people which described "sickness related behavioural dysfunction" (Bergner et al. 1981). The resulting statements were subjected to standard grouping and sorting techniques which yielded 312 unique items each of which described a sickness-related behavioural change. The prototype SIP, containing 312 items grouped into 14 categories of activity, was subsequently refined following a succession of field trials in 1973, 1974 and 1976, resulting in a final version with 136 statements and 12 categories. The SIP provides summary indices for physical, psychosocial and overall dysfunction as well as separate scores for the following 12 categories of activity: ambulation, mobility, body care and movement, social interaction, alertness behaviour, emotional behaviour, communication, sleep and rest, eating, work, home management, and recreation and pastimes. Only those statements which apply to respondents on the day of completion and are related to their health are endorsed, with simple dichotomous response categories of "Yes" or "No". Examples of statements include the following: "I walk shorter distance or stop to rest often" (Ambulation), "I am not doing any heavy work around the house that I usually do" (Home Management), "I am not doing any of my usual physical recreation or activities" (Recreation and Pastimes).

The instrument was scaled by its designers so that each item is weighted in terms of their relative degree of dysfunction. These weights were obtained using psychometric techniques of category-scaling which involved a total of 133 judges rating the relative "severity of dysfunction" of statements so that scale values could be assigned. The judging group comprised 108 randomly selected enrollees in a pre-paid health plan and 25 health care professionals and pre-professional students. Agreement among the judges was reported to be very high (Bergner 1988).

The overall score for the SIP is calculated by adding the scale values for each item checked across all categories and dividing the sum by the maximum possible dysfunction score for the SIP. This figure is then multiplied by 100 to give the overall SIP percentage score. The two sub-scores for physical and psychosocial dimensions are calculated by using a similar formula, but using only ambulation, bodycare and movement and mobility for the former, and social interaction, alertness behaviour, emotional behaviour, and communication for the latter. The other categories – sleep and rest, eating, work, home management, and recreation and pastimes – are each calculated separately as independent category scores. As discussed below, the components of these two sub-scores differ somewhat for the FLP as opposed to the SIP. The SIP can be self-completed or interviewer-administered, and takes between 20 to 30 minutes to complete.

Concerning reliability, Bergner et al. (1981), in a review of the development and final version of the SIP which involved extensive field trials, report high test-retest reliability ($r = 0.92$) and internal consistency ($r = 0.94$). The 1976 field trial also provided the basis to compare the reliability of three differing types of administration of the SIP: interviewer administered (I), interviewer delivered self-administration (ID) and mail-delivered self-administration (MD). High levels of test-retest reliability were found for I ($r = 0.97$) and ID ($r = 0.87$) formats (no retests on mail-delivered self-administration could be obtained), and no differences in overall mean scores between administrative types were found. Reproducibility of the individual items averaged 0.50, while for the overall score it was 0.92 (Bergner et al. 1981). Internal consistency was high (Cronbach's alpha 0.94). Internal consistency was also high for both Is ($r = 0.94$) and IDs ($r = 0.94$), but substantially lower for MDs ($r = 0.81$) (Bergner et al. 1981). Similarly, in a study of 79 outpatients with rheumatoid arthritis, Deyo et al. (1983) found SIP test-retest reliability to be 0.91 (Spearman's rank correlation) for 23 patients. Moreover, the SIP and its sub-scales were found to be more reliable than either the physician American Rheumatism Association's (ARA) functional ratings or patient self ratings.

SIP scores have been assessed for validity by comparing them with self reports of dysfunction and sickness; clinicians' reports of patient dysfunction and severity of illness; and with other measures of dysfunction and sickness such as the T_4 for hyperthyroidism, the Harris Analysis of Hip Function for hip replacement patients and the Activity Index for arthritic patients. Convergent and discriminant validity were evaluated using the multitrait-multimethod technique whilst clinical validity was assessed by determining the relationship between clinical measures of disease such as those mentioned above and SIP scores. The relationship between SIP scores and criterion measures were moderate to high and in the direction hypothesized. The results of field trials using the final version of the SIP showed higher correlations than were found using preliminary versions. For example, a correlation of 0.63 was found with a self assessment of sickness; 0.69 with a self assessment of dysfunction; 0.40 with clinicians' assessments of sickness; and finally, 0.50 with clinicians' assessments of dysfunction (Bergner et al. 1981). The rank correlation between the SIP and the Katz Index of Activities of Daily Living (IADL) was 0.46 in a 1974 field trial. However, as McDowell & Newell (1987) note, this relatively low correlation with the Katz IADL is due to the much broader coverage of the SIP and perhaps also from the low validity of the Katz instrument itself. The combined score for the five SIP categories that most clearly reflect ADL behaviours, however, correlated 0.64 (Bergner et al. 1976), while the correlation of the SIP with the National Health Interview Survey Index of Activity Limitation was 0.55 (Bergner et al. 1981).

Concerning its clinical validity, the SIP score correlated – 0.81 with the Harris Measure of Hip function for 15 hip replacement patients; 0.41

with Adjusted T_4 – a measure of thyroid function – in 14 hyperthyroid patients; and 0.66 with the Activity Index – a composite index of weighted values for morning stiffness, grip strength, sedimentation rate and joint involvement – in 15 rheumatoid arthritis patients (Bergner et al. 1981). In another study, Deyo and colleagues (1983), reported correlations between the SIP and a range of indicators of disease severity for 79 patients with RA. Scores on the SIP or its sub-scales were found to yield higher correlations than clinical ratings of ARA functional class or patient self ratings of function with hematocrit, sedimentation rate (ESR), grip strength, morning stiffness, duration of RA, anatomic stage, employment status and psychiatric status. A regular progression was also found between the mean SIP score and physical dimension score (but not the psychosocial dimension score) with increasing ARA rank. Moreover, Deyo et al. found that the validity of the SIP appeared to be maintained with repeated administrations; no trend was detected towards deterioration of the validity coefficients with repeated administration. More recent evidence regarding the SIP's strong validity properties has been provided by Read and his colleagues (1987) in their evaluation of the General Health Rating Index (GHRI), the Quality of Well-Being Scale (QWB) and the Sickness Impact Profile (SIP). These and other findings attest to the reliability and validity of the SIP and to its utility as a supplement to more traditional measures of chronic disease outcome.

In the US, a Chicano-Spanish version of the SIP has been developed and described by Gilson et al. (1980), whilst de Bruin and colleagues (1993), in their recent review of the SIP, found seven translations in Europe: into British, Swedish, German, French (two translations), Danish, Norwegian and Dutch.

The British version of the SIP, the Functional Limitations Profile (FLP), was developed by Patrick and his colleagues at St Thomas's Hospital London for their community survey of disability in Lambeth (Patrick & Peach 1989). Wherever necessary, items were re-worded in order to make them more meaningful to the British populace. The FLP was tested in a pilot study using general practice patients in Kingston-upon-Thames (Patrick et al. 1982, Patrick & Peach 1989). A partial rescaling was also conducted using a sample of individuals from Lambeth as judges in order to investigate possible cultural differences between British and American populations. The Lambeth FLP values were highly predictive of the Seattle SIP values indicating that the judges gave remarkably similar ratings to the items (Patrick et al. 1985, Patrick &

Peach 1989). Consequently, the differences between the SIP and FLP are minimal.

As with the SIP, respondents are asked whether or not each statement describes them today and, if so, whether this is due to their health. If this is so, then the scale weight attached to that item contributes to the respondents disability scores. Again, as with the SIP, scores are calculated for each category by adding together the scale weights for each item checked, dividing by the maximum possible category score and then multiplying by 100 to obtain the percentage FLP category score. A similar procedure is used to obtain the overall FLP score. In contrast to the SIP, however, the categories that comprise the dimension scores are slightly different. Physical disability is comprised of each item ticked within the ambulation, bodycare and movement, mobility and household management categories, whilst the psychosocial dimension score is composed of items ticked within the recreation and pastimes, social interaction, emotions, alertness, sleep and rest categories. Unlike its American counterpart, the FLP has been much less extensively tried and tested and few studies exist to date concerning its use and application in the UK. As Bowling (1991) notes, the FLP requires far more testing for reliability and validity before it can truly be considered the UK alternative to the SIP.

Applications of the SIP and FLP in research: the case of chronic respiratory illness

The SIP has been used extensively in a wide range of studies and across many different patient groups (mostly chronic) mainly in the USA, but also in the UK and other parts of the world. For example, it has been used to good effect in the following areas: cardiac arrest and cardiac rehabilitation (Bergner et al. 1985, Ott et al. 1983); angina (Vandenburg 1988, Fletcher et al. 1988); heart transplantation evaluations (Wenger et al. 1984); head injury (Temkin et al. 1988, 1989); Alzheimers-type dementia (Krenz et al. 1988); chronic lung disease (McSweeney et al. 1980, 1982, Prigatano et al. 1984, Bergner et al. 1988, Jones 1991, 1992); cancer (Greenwald 1987); end stage renal disease (Hart & Evans 1987); hyperthyroidism (Bergner et al. 1981); rheumatoid arthritis (Bergner et al. 1981, Deyo et al. 1982, 1983, Deyo 1988); hip replacement (Bergner et al.

1981); total joint replacement (Liang et al. 1985); low back pain (Roland & Morris 1983, Deyo & Diehl 1983; Deyo 1986; Follick et al. 1985); chronic pain (Watt-Watson & Graydon, 1989); dental conditions (Reisine et al. 1989); speech pathology (Pollard et al. 1976); women with urinary incontinence (Hunskaar & Vinsnes 1991); psoriasis (Finlay et al. 1990); and in assessing the functional status of older patients with chronic illness (Goldsmith & Brodwick 1989). The advantage of this wide applicability, of course, as Bowling (1991) notes, is that scores from many different population groups are readily available for comparison using a standard instrument.

In contrast, as mentioned above, the UK version of the SIP, the FLP, has been much less extensively used. For example, it has recently been used to good effect in a longitudinal study of disability in Lambeth where it proved to be a far more sensitive and comprehensive measure than the 1969 OPCS/NS instrument (Patrick & Peach 1989). It has also recently been used in studies of patients with rheumatoid arthritis (Fitzpatrick et al. 1988a, 1988b, 1992, Jenkinson et al. 1991), and a study of the quality of life of people with chronic obstructive airways disease (COAD) (Williams & Bury 1989a, 1989b, Williams 1990, 1993).

Rather than attempting to provide a comprehensive review of studies which have used the SIP and the FLP, this section of the chapter focuses more specifically upon the use of these instruments in relation to chronic respiratory illness, as an illustrative example of the application, performance and utility of the SIP and FLP in empirical research. Reviews of a more general nature can be found elsewhere (Bergner et al. 1981, Bergner 1988, Wenger et al. 1984, McDowell & Newell 1987, Walker & Rosser 1988, Bowling 1991, de Bruin et al. 1993).

A major large-scale American study which utilized the SIP was the Nocturnal Oxygen Therapy Trial (NOTT). This was a multi-site collaborative study which was designed to compare the effectiveness of nocturnal or continuous oxygen therapy for patients with chronic obstructive pulmonary disease (COPD: chronic bronchitis and emphysema) with notable hypoxaemia ($PaO_2 < 60\,mm\,Hg$) (McSweeny et al. 1980, 1982). The baseline study provided the opportunity to describe in detail the type and level of dysfunction experienced by COPD patients, as well as the relationship between the SIP and several other physical and neuropsychological measures. In addition, other measures, such as the Minnesota Multiphasic Personality Inventory (MMPI), the Profile of Mood States (POMS), and the Katz Adjustment Scale (KAS) (completed by relatives), comprised a comprehensive battery of tests designed to examine the quality of life of COPD patients.

The results of comparisons between COPD patients and control subjects showed that the quality of life of these patients was impaired on all dimensions. Scores on the SIP indicated that COPD patients experience both considerable levels and a breadth of dysfunction. For example, the mean overall SIP for these patients was found to be approximately 25%, and COPD patients generally displayed a much higher percentage of impairment across SIP categories than the control group. Although displaying the highest dysfunction score, the employment category was the only one which was not significantly different between COPD patients and the control group, due, the investigators claim, to the fact that both groups contained many elderly retired persons. The areas of functioning most severely affected on the SIP were recreation and pastimes, home management and sleep and rest. Indeed, the SIP results suggest reductions of between 40% and 50% in pleasurable activities. In contrast, eating and communication appeared to be only moderately affected by the disease (McSweeny et al. 1980, 1982). McSweeny et al. noted, however, that there was considerable variability in the life quality of these COPD patients as measured by the SIP and other instruments.

Prigatano et al. (1984) also used the SIP with COPD patients with mild hypoxaemia. Generally, their findings were similar to those obtained by McSweeny et al. (1980, 1982) with severly hypoxaemic patients, although, as might be expected, the degree of impairment was proportionately less. For example, a reduction of between 30% and 40% in pleasurable activities was seen in these mildly hypoxaemic patients on the SIP, compared to McSweeny et al.'s finding of between 40% and 50% in severely hypoxaemic patients. However, in contrast to McSweeny et al.'s study, Prigatano et al. did find significant differences in SIP employment category scores between COPD patients and controls.

McSweeny et al. (1982) also went on to examine the relationship between life quality, as represented by overall SIP scores, and various socio-physical and neuropsychological variables. The SIP score was found to correlate quite poorly with the physiological measures normally used to assess the severity of COPD. For example, Pearson's correlation (r) between the SIP and a severity of disease index (which included forced expiratory volume, maximum exercise tolerance, resting heart rate, oxygen saturation before exercise and pulmonary artery pressure) was only 0.17 ($p < 0.02$); -0.16 ($p < 0.04$) with a cardiac index; and -0.33 ($p < 0.01$)

with a measure of maximum workload during exercise. Correlations of SIP scores with various neuropsychological measures were also only moderate, ranging from $r = 0.34$ ($p < 0.01$) to $r = 0.45$ ($p < 0.01$). However, as McSweeny et al. point out, although these relationships between the SIP and medicophysiological variables are only modest, entry criteria for the NOTT only permitted COPD patients with a restricted range of pulmonary function to enter the study, thereby decreasing the likelihood of high correlations.

An exploratory multiple regression procedure was also used to examine the combined contribution of age, social class, neuropsychological functioning and psychological functioning to life quality as measured by the SIP. The specific variables regressed against the SIP overall score were age, socio-economic status, a global neuropsychological rating and a severity of disease index. The resulting function was highly significant, although the multiple correlation produced was moderate, accounting for 25% of the variance in quality of life as measured by the SIP. All variables contributed significantly to the overall relationship with the SIP. Age (partial correlation $r = 0.31$), socio-economic status (partial correlation $r = 0.26$), and neuropsychological functioning (partial correlation $r = 0.22$), seemed to be relatively more important in relation to quality of life than pathophysiological status (partial correlation $r = 0.15$) for this particular group of patients.

Prigatano et al.'s (1984) study lends further support to McSweeny et al.'s results, as well as producing some other interesting findings. In particular, Prigatano et al. found that COPD patients' quality of life, as measured on the SIP, was negatively related to smoking history, but not to recent life changes. In addition, Prigatano et al. found that neuropsychological functioning, exercise capability and pulmonary function variables displayed a stronger relationship to physical aspects of quality of life than to psychosocial aspects of quality of life, as measured on the SIP. In contrast, mood and emotional functioning measured on the MMPI and the POMS were more strongly related to the psychosocial aspects of quality of life on the SIP. These findings demonstrate the applicability and relevance of the SIP as a quality of life measure in COPD. In the NOTT trial, however, no significant differences were found in SIP scores between the two treatment groups at the end of the trial. However, this should not necessarily be seen as a weakness of the SIP, as similarly no clear-cut physiological differences were found which completely explained the increased mortality of those on nocturnal oxygen therapy.

Broadly similar results were obtained by Williams and Bury (1989a, 1989b, Williams 1990), in a study of the quality of life of 92 outpatients with chronic obstructive airways disease (COAD) using the FLP. As in McSweeny et al.'s (1982) study, COAD patients were found to suffer considerable limitations across a broad range of categories and areas of life. Again, areas found to be particularly affected included household management (men tending to score lower on this domain than women, t-test $p < 0.0001$), ambulation, sleep and rest, recreation and pastimes and work (men tending to score higher in this domain than women, t-test $p < 0.03$). A profile of the mean FLP scores is given in Table 8.1.

Table 8.1 Mean ranked FLP category scores in chronic obstructive airways disease (COAD).

FLP category	Mean %
1. Work	42
2. Recreation and Pastimes	40
3. Household Management	35
4. Sleep and Rest	32
5. Ambulation	28
6. Alertness	25
7. Mobility	23
8. Social Interaction	20
9. Emotion	20
10. Bodycare and Movement	15
11. Communication	9
12. Eating	5
Physical Dimension	20
Psychosocial	19
Overall	22

Note; In the Lambeth disability study, community controls (i.e. men and women in the following two age bands: 25–64, 65–77 yrs) scored less than 6 per cent on all FLP categories (Patrick & Peach 1989).

The various measures of dyspnoea included in the study all correlated well with one another and with the FLP physical disability dimension score as expected: for example, a high negative correlation of -0.90 ($p < 0.001$) was found between the oxygen cost diagram (OCD) and FLP physical disability dimension score (the negative correlation implying that the lesser the magnitude of the task provoking breathlessness, the higher the FLP physical disability score), which dropped to -0.62 ($p < 0.001$) after controlling for spirometry, age and psychological distress. Statistically significant differences were also found with respect to mean FLP physical disability scores across MRC breathlessness gradings, suggesting some degree of convergent validity. These findings are shown in Table 8.2.

Table 8.2 The relationship between FLP physical disability scores and breathlessness in COAD (using one-way ANOVA and the Scheffe multiple comparisons test).

	Mean global FLP physical disability	Fletcher (MRC) breathlessness grading		
		2	3	4 5
Fletcher (MRC)	2 7.7			
breathlessness	3 12.7	*		
grading	4 20.3	*	*	
	5 26.2	*	*	*

* Denotes significance at the p < 0.5 level.

These results serve to highlight the very close relationship which exists between breathlessness and the degree of physical disability experienced, and confirms the suggestion that dyspnoea is one of the most distressing and disabling symptoms of COAD (Rosser et al. 1983, Lane 1878, Jones 1988).

In addition, the FLP physical disability dimension score was also found to correlate 0.44 with age (p < 0.001) and 0.60 (p < 0.001) with the General Health Questionnaire (GHQ-12). However, as in McSweeny et al.'s (1980, 1982) study, only moderate correlations were found to exist between the spirometric measures of lung function (FEV 1 % of predicted normal) and the FLP physical disability score (−0.38 p < 0.001), and the amount of variance explained was only 14%. A summary of these correlations is presented in Table 8.3.

Finally, Jones and colleagues (1989), in another interesting recent study, investigated the relationship between the SIP, respiratory symptoms, physiological measures and mood in patients with chronic airflow limitation. The patients in this study had less severe lung disease than those in the NOTT study. This was the result of a deliberate intention to cover a wider range of disease severity in order to permit satisfactory correlation between variables. As expected, the SIP scores were found to be lower than in those previously reported studies in which the patients had greater physiological disturbance, but the profile of the different SIP

Table 8.3 Summary of zero–order correlations between FLP physical disability scores and other clinical variables in COAD.

	Global FLP physical disability score
1. Spirometry	−0.38*
2. Dyspnoea	−0.90*[1]
3. Age	0.44*
4. Psychological distress	0.60*

* Significant at the (p < 0.001) level.
[1] Partial correlation controlling for spirometry, age and psychological distress −0.62 (p < 0.001).

categories was found to be similar. SIP scores were also found to be considerably higher in those who wheezed everyday compared with those who did not do so (p < 0.0005). The total SIP score was found to exhibit a high negative correlation with the six minute walking distance test (6MWD) r = −0.64 (p < 0.0001); one which was stronger than with any of the physiological measures used to assess such patients. In addition to the correlation between the total SIP and the 6MWD test, significant correlations were also observed with a number of other variables, both objective and subjective. For example, FVC (% of predicted normal) accounted for 13.5% (p < 0.001) of the variance in SIP scores, 6MWD 41% (p < 0.001) of the variance, and anxiety and depression scores measured on the Hospital Anxiety and Depression Questionnaire (HAD) accounted for 26.1% (p < 0.001) and 38.4% (p < 0.001) of the variance respectively. In short, the 6MWD and the scores for anxiety and depression were found to correlate more strongly with SIP scores than the best spirometric measures and measures of physiological functioning.

Multiple regression against the total SIP score showed that there was no effect of FVC on the SIP score after removal of the variance due to 6MWD. In contrast, anxiety, depression and MRC dyspnoea scores each had a significant effect on the total SIP score (p < 0.001 in each case) which was independent of the effect of 6MWD. Indeed a multiple regression equation containing 6MWD, depression score, and MRC dyspnoea score accounted for 62% of the variance in the total SIP score. As in Williams and Bury's (1989a, 1989b, Williams 1990) study, the total SIP score was also found to increase with increasing MRC dyspnoea grades (ANOVA p < 0.0001). The total SIP scores for the respective MRC dyspnoea grades were as follows: Grade 1, 3.9 (4.6 SD); Grade 2, 3.5 (4.1 SD); Grade

3, 7.7 (6.0 SD); Grade 4, 12.1 (7.7 SD); Grade 5, 17.6 (8.9 SD). Age, sex and response to bronchodilator were not found to be correlated with SIP scores. On the basis of these findings, Jones and his colleagues conclude that the SIP provides a valid measure of general health in a population of patients with chronic airflow limitation.

In summary, the SIP is a carefully developed, extensively tested, reliable and valid instrument, which has been used in a variety of settings for a number of different purposes, and, as this example of COAD serves to illustrate, is versatile enough to be broadly applicable to a wide range of patient groups and illness conditions. Moreover, the high degree of convergence between the findings of these studies of COPD/COAD provides further support for the external validity of the SIP. In this respect, the SIP may indeed serve as a standard against which to judge other instruments. Yet despite this, both the SIP and the FLP do have certain limitations. Hence it is to a consideration of some of these limitations that this chapter now turns.

Limitations of the SIP and the FLP

In a much cited paper on health status indicators, Jette (1980) criticises the SIP for the following reasons:

> First, there is a lack of measurement sensitivity; for instance, the SIP focuses on ability vs inability to perform activities, thus neglecting the range of performance in between (e.g. "I am not going into town"; or, "I am not doing heavy work around the house"). Second, it uses multiple functional activities within the same question which may be performed at different levels of function (e.g. "I have given up taking care of personal or household business affairs, for example, paying bills, banking, working on a budget"; or "I have difficulty doing housework, for example, turning faucets, kitchen gadgets, sewing, carpentry"). Finally, it provides limited attention to the more subjective components of performance, such as pain or trouble. (Jette 1980: 571).

The points Jette raises are certainly important, particularly the last, although the SIP does, of course, include behavioural statements which relate to these more subjective components of performance such as pain (e.g. in the emotion category: "I keep rubbing or holding areas of my body that hurt or are uncomfortable"). Yet beyond these points, a number of other issues also emerge. Perhaps the first issue concerns the range of possible scores. As discussed earlier, with the exception of the employment category, the SIP/FLP is designed to provide percentage disability scores ranging from 0 to 100%. In reality, however, this proves impossible in the majority of cases due to the fact that various statements logically preclude others. In the ambulation category, for example, the statement "I do not walk at all" logically precludes the statement "I walk more slowly". Similarly, the statement "I do not use stairs at all" logically precludes the affirmation of the statement "I go up and down stairs more slowly". Consequently, it becomes logically impossible to affirm all the statements in the ambulation category, thus making the claim that scores range from 0 to 100% incorrect. Moreover, as Jones (1991) reports, in a study of 152 patients with moderately severe chronic obstructive airways disease (COAD), 20% of the items in the SIP were left completely unchecked by every patient, whilst approximately a quarter of the questionnaire items accounted for two-thirds of the total number of positive responses. Consequently, the overall effect of this "is to produce very low scores even in patients who have moderate levels of disability" (Jones 1991: 679).

A second, related, issue concerns the fact that, due to certain statements logically precluding others, the potential arises for those who are severely disabled to end up having somewhat lower category scores than those who are less severely disabled. For example, a paraplegic person would affirm the following statements "I do not walk at all" (FLP weight 126), "I only get about in a wheelchair" (FLP weight 121) and "I do not use stairs at all" (FLP weight 106). As discussed above, these statements logically preclude others, for one cannot walk more slowly and not walk at all, or use stairs more slowly and not use stairs at all. In contrast, an arthritic person who can still walk and negotiate stairs, albeit with difficulty, may affirm the following combination of statements: "I walk shorter distances or often stop for a rest" (FLP weight 054), "I walk more slowly" (FLP weight 039), "I walk by myself but with some difficulty, for example, I limp" (FLP weight 071), "I do not walk up or down hill" (FLP weight 064), "I go up and down stairs more slowly" (FLP weight 062) and finally, "I only use stairs with a physical aid, for example, a handrail" (FLP weight 082). This results in a total FLP score of 353 for the paraplegic person and a score of 372 for the arthritic respondent: giving FLP disability scores for the ambulation category of 35% and 37% respectively. Thus although more severe items carry more weight, certain combinations of more severe items logically preclude the affirmation of larger combinations of less severe items, resulting, potentially at least, in a higher disability score for the less disabled.

Thirdly, in the light of these points, there is, in fact, good reason to dispense with the weighting of the FLP altogether. As de Bruin et al. (1993) have pointed out, methodological literature suggests that nominal weighting, as used in the scaling of the SIP, has its greatest effect on the ordering of individuals in composite scores when there is considerable variation in item weights, when there is little inter-item correlation amongst the components, and when there are a small number of component parts. The SIP, in contrast, has a relatively large number of items (n = 136), and has been developed with a concern for internal consistency (i.e. high inter-item correlations). Consequently:

> . . . the differences between item weights in the SIP are too small to have any important impact upon either the total or dimension score. Therefore, the rank order of persons in a distribution of weighted scores will be almost identical to the rank order of the distribution of unweighted scores. An alternative is not to use weights but simply to add the number of items checked. In a sense, this procedure uses weights of 1 for every item. This is the simplest procedure. (de Bruin et al. 1993: 1011).

In a recent empirical investigation of these issues, Jenkinson and his colleagues (1991) administered the NHP and the FLP to 101 rheumatoid arthritis (RA) patients on two separate occasions separated by three months. Change scores were calculated using both the weighted scores and also by simply summing dichotomous scores expressed as a percentage. Results were found to be strikingly similar, with the resultant correlations never lower than 0.96 (p < 0.0001) for NHP scores, and 0.93 (p < 0.0001) for FLP scores. Consequently it was suggested that, due to insufficient weight variance, these questionnaires may give equally valid results with unweighted scores. Similarly, Fitzpatrick et al. (1988) suggest that, in view of the comparable performances of the FLP and the HAQ found in their study, nothing appeared to be gained in terms of precision by the use of weighted items over the simpler ordinal assumptions of the HAQ.

A fourth, crucial, issue, and one which has received relatively little attention to date, concerns the "sensitivity" or "responsiveness" of the instrument to the detection of change over time and its clinical significance. As we have seen, whilst a great deal of attention has been paid to establishing the instrument's reliability and validity, surprisingly little work has been directed towards investigating its responsiveness and its clinical significance. Yet this is crucial for an evaluative instrument such as the SIP/FLP. As de Bruin et al. state:

> The SIP is meant to be used in longitudinal designs. In most studies, however, it was evaluated as a descriptive or predictive instrument to discriminate between or within groups in cross-sectional research designs. A discriminative index should have a good reliability and should detect differences between individuals at one moment in time. An evaluative instrument should detect clinically important changes over time. Little is known about the ability of the SIP to detect those changes. (1993: 1010).

Several methods have been proposed in order to assess and quantify responsiveness (Deyo 1988), but as yet no standard method has been found and no criterion is generally accepted. Only in a few more recent studies has the responsiveness of the SIP/FLP been assessed.

Liang and colleagues (1985), for example, conducted a comparative study of the measurement efficiency and sensitivity of five health status instruments which were each administered to 50 arthritis patients before and after they had total joint arthroplasty. Marked improvements in pain levels and functional performance were found 3 months after discharge. Using the FSI as the criterion measure against which to assess the relative efficiency (RE) of the other instruments (i.e. the FSI's RE = 1.00), the AIMS, FSI and the SIP were all approximately equal in terms of their efficiency in detecting changes in mobility scores, whilst the HAQ and IWB were only about half as efficient. Of the three measures used for pain assessment, the AIMS was 79% efficient relative to the FSI in detecting change, whereas the HAQ was only 57% efficient. Regarding the detection of changes in social function, the AIMS was inefficient (RE = 0.18) compared to the FSI, whilst the relative efficiency of the other instruments was between 0.54 for the IWB and 0.74 for the SIP. Finally, regarding the global indices of functional impairments, the FSI (RE = 1.00) and HAQ (RE = 1.15) performed equally, but they were less than one-third as efficient as the SIP

(RE = 3.51), the AIMS (RE = 4.12) and the IWB (RE = 7.50). Inter-instrument correlations of functional change were generally lower than for the cross-sectional pre-operative data. However, in this study, no single instrument consistently out-performed the others, and the SIP appeared to be relatively efficient at detecting change.

In another comparative study of health status measures in rheumatoid arthritis, Fitzpatrick et al. (1988b) assessed 105 RA patients on two separate occasions separated by a 15 month period by means of the ARA functional scale, the Malaya and Mace Index (which comprises six measures (ESR, Hb, grip strength, an articular index, morning stiffness and a pain scale), the HAQ and the FLP. Of these patients, 33 per cent were found to have clinically changed across the study period in terms of the ARA scale. On both occasions cross-sectional correlations were strongest between the two health status instruments (HAQ and the FLP) and grip strength (HAQ t1 – 0.73 and t2 – 0.68; FLP t1 – 0.66 and t2 – 0.67) and the Ritchie articular index (HAQ t1 0.69 and t2 0.58; total FLP t1 – 0.62 and t2 – 0.55). The sensitivity and the specificity of these two instruments in relation to clinical change was also assessed and, as Fitzpatrick et al. state on the basis of their findings: "It may be said that, at best, the two instruments perform moderately well as measures of change over time". Overall HAQ and FLP scores achieved similarly modest levels of sensitivity and specificity, and neither instrument was markedly superior. It was also found that the FLP appeared to be consistently more sensitive and specific in relation to deterioration compared to improvement. These results are similar to those obtained by Deyo and Inui (1984) with the SIP in a sample of outpatients with RA.

Finally, in another more recent investigation, Fitzpatrick et al. (1992) assessed the sensitivity to change over time of the AIMS, the HAQ, the NHP, and the FLP in relation to 101 patients with RA across a three month period. For all dimensions of health status measured, the magnitude of change varied considerably according to the instrument. The maximum range in effect size – calculated as mean change divided by baseline standard deviation of the variable – was for the social scales (AIMS 0.06, NHP 0.24, FLP 0.60) and no single instrument seemed consistently to show the most change across all the dimensions assessed.

In summary, the issue of the responsiveness of the SIP/FLP seems to have been a relatively neglected area to date, and no firm conclusions can, as yet, be drawn. However, in tests conducted to date, the SIP/FLP appears to perform moderately well and to compare favourably with other measures of health status, although there is a suggestion that it may be less sensitive to improvement than deterioration. However, further investigation into this issue is needed.

The fifth issue concerns the nature and meaning of overall scores. As Hunt et al. (1985) suggest, overall scores may be arrived at via many different routes and are composed of logically incompatible domains such as ambulation and eating, making them at best meaningless and at worst redundant. Moreover, maximum possible SIP/FLP category scores differ. Consequently their respective contributions to the overall score vary, despite the fact that their percentage disability scores may be similar. For example, a 25% body care and movement score contributes 4.85% to the total FLP score, whilst a 25% sleep and rest score only contributes 1.78% to the total FLP score. The rationale for this, of course, is that there are more items in the bodycare and movement category (n = 23) than in the sleep and rest category (n = 7). Consequently to obtain a 25% score, for example, more items have to be checked in the former than the latter category, and hence this is reflected in the overall score. This may be a reasonable enough argument, yet it does mean that categories, implicitly or by default, are weighted in terms of their maximum potential contributions to the overall FLP score. Hence we get the following pattern of maximum potential contributions to the total FLP score: ambulation 10.14%, bodycare and movement 19.42%, mobility 7.33%, household management 6.90%, recreation and pastimes 3.86%, social interaction 12.99%, emotion 6.99%, alertness 7.17%, sleep and rest 7.17%, eating 7.11%, communication 6.90%, and work 5.24%.

The sixth issue concerns the practicality of using the SIP and the FLP, and the rationale for modifying or shortening these instruments. The SIP and the FLP are lengthy instruments to administer and the greater amount of information they provide has to be weighed against the shorter length and time needed to administer other instruments such as the NHP (Hunt et al. 1985, 1986), which has only 38 items in part I, intended to measure subjective health status, and the SF-36 questionnaire (Ware & Sherbourne 1992), with 36 items. Indeed, Bowling (1991) reports that the FLP was rejected for use in evaluations of heart-disease treatment programmes in the UK on the grounds of its length, and instead, the more concise NHP was selected in preference (Buxton 1983, O'Brien 1988). However, the NHP is not without its own limitations, particularly the rather extreme nature and severity of the items it contains (Kind & Carr-Hill 1987).

In an evaluative study of three health status measures – the General Health Rating Index (GHRI), the Quality of Well-Being Scale (QWB) and the Sickness Impact Profile (SIP), Read et al. (1987) assessed the practicality of each measure in terms of the degree of interviewer training required, administration time, and respondent burden. They found that each instrument was practical for use in their research, with some noteworthy exceptions. In terms of interviewer training time they found that the instruments varied considerably from 1 to 2 hours for the GHRI, 1 week for the SIP, to 1 to 2 weeks for the QWB. Once trained, however, their interviewers reported that the SIP and the QWB were roughly equivalent in terms of difficulty of administration (moderate-high). Neither was particularly burdensome, although the lengthy sequence of questions in the SIP became somewhat tedious with repetition. All three instruments were found to be acceptable to respondents and they rarely voiced complaints about individual items or difficulty. The administration time between instruments was, however, found to be significantly different rising from a mean of 11.4 (4.4 SD) minutes for the GHRI, to 18.2 (9.4) minutes for the QWB, and 22.4 (8.7 SD) minutes for the SIP.

In another study, Deyo et al. (1989) found that only 2% of patients' reactions to the SIP were negative (71% positive, 27% neutral). Typical responses included the following: "did not understand some of words", "too long", "did not apply to me". Filling out the SIP was not found to cause distress or discomfort for most respondents (97%). Critical comments, however, included the following: "too many questions and very stressful", "little negative" (de Bruin et al. 1993).

However, although comments on the use of the SIP have generally been favourable, the length and the time required to complete the SIP/FLP raise important questions about their modification to shorter versions. The categorical nature of these instruments, and the well-defined nature of the areas of activity covered, certainly make them amenable to modification. In this respect, several researchers have attempted to use parts of the SIP/FLP in their studies, and in general the modified or shortened version of the SIP/FLP seems robust enough to have served these researchers purposes (de Bruin et al. 1993). Roland & Morris (1983), for example, extracted a 24-item version from the FLP: the Roland scale, which was designed for patients with acute low back pain. In terms of its correlations with physical measures of disease severity and with overall SIP scores (Deyo 1986), this scale appears as least as valid as lengthier scales (de Bruin et al. 1993). Similarly, in Fitzpatrick et al. (1988) study of RA, the additional information which the FLP provided compared to the HAQ did not increase the size of the correlations with conventional measures, nor did it add to the sensitivity to change provided by the physical scale of the FLP alone. In summary, these and other findings suggest that a modified or shortened version of the SIP/FLP is possible. Most of these modifications appear to discriminate between levels of health, evaluate patients responses to treatment and predict future states (de Bruin et al. 1993).

Finally, a more general issue concerns the meaning and interpretation of SIP/FLP scores. In addition to the issues raised earlier about the clinical significance of these scores, little attention has been devoted to attempting to understand the precise meaning and location of these scores in the context of people's daily lives and social circumstances. The relevance of these issues for interpreting SIP/FLP scores is clearly illustrated by the following examples; the first relating to mobility scores and the second to scores in the household management category. Responses to statements in these categories may be answered quite differently by respondents with comparable levels of disability, according to their particular social circumstances and resources. For example, regarding mobility, one man may previously have travelled to work via public transport until, eventually, his health became progressively worse and he decided to use his car instead. However, a second man, in contrast, who does not have access to a car, is left with little option but to struggle on using public transport in order to get to his place of work. In this example, the first respondent affirms the statement "I do not use public transport now" whilst the second does not do so. Does this then mean that the first man experiences more "behavioural dysfunction" regarding public transport than his equally disabled counterpart? Similarly, with respect to household management, a married woman whose health has deteriorated, finds shopping a real struggle. Consequently her husband now does it for her. In contrast, a comparably disabled single, widowed, or divorced woman who lives alone but does not want to be a burden upon anybody, continues to struggle with her own shopping, despite the fact that it leaves her drained and exhausted. Again, the first woman affirms the statement "I do not do any of the shopping that I would usually do" whilst the second woman does not do so. Are we, once again, to assume that the first woman experiences more "behavioural dysfunction" regarding shopping than her equally disabled counterpart?

This, it should be said, is not a specific criticism of either the SIP or the FLP. Rather, it represents a more general point regarding the failure to interpret and locate the meaning of these statements and scores within the context of people's daily lives. As such it draws attention to a very different type of "validity" with respect to these scores and their interpretation. A broadly similar point is made by de Bruin et al. (1993) who, at the end of their review of the SIP, mention the lack of research concerning the theoretical relevance of SIP scores.

Conclusions: towards a balance sheet

Measuring health is a complex goal: the epistemic gap between concepts and indicators is nowhere more acutely felt than in relation to the measurement of health. This, however, is not to say that we should give up hope; rather considerable progress in health status measurement has been made in recent years, and the search for an ever more perfect "mousetrap" (Liang et al. 1982) continues. This chapter has been concerned with discussing and evaluating one such attempt: namely, the Sickness Impact Profile and its UK equivalent, the Functional Limitations Profile.

Given these inevitable constraints, it is clear that the SIP represents one of the most sophisticated and comprehensive attempts to date to assess health status. Moreover, it has been extensively tested and has been shown to be a reliable and valid instrument. In this respect, as mentioned earlier, the SIP may well become the standard against which other health status measures are judged (McDowell & Newell 1987). In contrast, the FLP requires far more testing for reliability and validity before it can be considered the UK alternative to the SIP (Bowling 1991), although work of this nature is beginning to accumulate.

Yet despite these positive features, it is clear that both the SIP and FLP suffer from certain limitations. As we have seen, chief amongst these are the problems concerning the range of possible scores, insufficient variation in scale weights resulting in dichotomous scores yielding similar data, the lack of research regarding the responsiveness and the clinical significance of their scores, doubts concerning the meaningfulness of overall scores comprised from logically incompatible domains, the practicality of using these instruments in terms of time and length, and hence the rationale for their modification, and finally, the more general problem of the meaning, interpretation and significance of these scores when divorced from the context of people's daily lives.

This suggests that researchers should carefully weigh up the pros and cons of using these instruments and assess their suitability for the particular study in question. Certainly, the SIP and the FLP provide a broad and detailed range of information which, as Deyo et al. (1983) suggest, may represent a useful supplement to more traditional measures of (chronic) disease outcome. Yet this has to be weighed against, for instance, the length and the time taken to complete these instrument, or the need to modify them.

Health status measurement is a burgeoning industry, and a proliferation of measures now exists, including the NHP (Hunt et al. 1986), the QWB (Kaplan & Anderson 1988), and the SF-36 (Ware & Sherbourne 1992). Given the "state of the art" of health status measurement, the SIP appears to compare favourably with most instruments to date. However, whether it will be "eclipsed" in time by the development of other instruments which, with ever more precision, seek to grasp that most elusive and nebulous of concepts "health", remains to be seen.

Functional Limitations Profile questionnaire

The following are statements about your current health and how it may influence your everyday life. Please answer "Yes" if an item applies to you today and you feel that this is due to your health. Otherwise answer "No".

Alertness

I am confused and start to do more than one thing at a time.

I have more minor accidents; for example, I drop things, I trip and fall, I bump into things.

I react slowly to things that are said or done.

I do not finish things I start.

I have difficulty reasoning and solving problems, for example, making plans, making decisions, learning new things.

I sometimes get confused, for example, I do not know where I am, who is around or what day it is.

I forget a lot, for example, things that happened recently, where I put things, or to keep appointments.

I do not keep my attention on any activity for long.

I make more mistakes than usual.

I have difficulty doing things which involve thought and concentration.

Housework

I only do housework or work around the house for short periods of time or I rest often.

I do less of the daily household chores than I would normally do.

I do not do any of the daily household chores that I would usually do.

I do not do any of the maintenance or repair work that I would usually do in my home or garden.

I do not do any of the shopping that I would usually do.

I do not do any of the cleaning that I would usually do.

I have difficulty using my hands; for example, turning taps, using kitchen gadgets, sewing or doing repairs.

I do not do any of the clothes washing that I would usually do.

I do not do heavy work around the house.

I have given up taking care of personal or household business affairs; for example, paying bills, banking or doing household accounts.

Mobility

I only get about in one building.

I stay in one room.

I stay in bed more.

I stay in bed most of the time.

I do not use public transport now.

I stay at home most of the time.

I only go out if there is a lavatory nearby.

I do not go into the shopping centre.

I only stay away from home for short periods.

I do not get about in the dark or in places that are not lit unless I have someone to help.

Bodycare and movement

Difficult movements like getting in or out of bed I do with help.

I do not get in and out of bed or chairs without the help of a personal or mechanical aid.

I only stand for short periods of time.

I do not keep my balance.

I move my hands or fingers with some difficulty or limitation.

I only stand up with someone's help.

I kneel, stoop or bend down only by holding onto something.

I am in a restricted position all the time.

I am very clumsy.

I get in and out of bed or chairs by grasping something for support or by using a stick or walking frame.

I stay lying down most of the time.

I change position frequently.

I hold onto something to move myself around in bed.

I do not bath myself completely, for example, I need help with bathing.

I do not bath myself at all but am bathed by someone else.

I use a bedpan with help.

I have trouble putting on my shoes, socks or stockings.

I do not have control of my bladder.

I do not fasten my clothing; for example, I require assistance with buttons, zips or shoelaces.

I spend most of the time partly dressed or in pyjamas.

I do not have control of my bowels.

I dress myself, but do so very slowly.
I only get dressed with someone's help.

Sleep and rest
I spend much of the day lying down to rest.
I sit for much of the day.
I sleep or doze most of the time – day and night.
I lie down to rest more often during the day.
I sit around half asleep.
I sleep less at night, for example I wake up easily, I don't fall asleep for a
    long time, or I keep waking up.
I sleep or doze more during the day.

Recreation and pastimes
I spend shorter periods of time on my hobbies and recreation.
I go out to enjoy myself less often.
I am cutting down on some of my usual inactive pastimes, for example, I
    watch TV less, play cards less or read less.
I am not doing any of my usual inactive pastimes, for example, I do not
    watch TV, play cards or read.
I am doing more inactive pastimes instead of my other usual activities.
I take part in fewer community activities.
I am cutting down on some of my usual physical recreation or more
    active pastimes.
I am not doing any of my usual physical recreation or more active pas-
    times.

Social interactions
I go out to visit people less often.
I do not go out to visit people at all.
I show less interest in other people's problems, for example, I don't lis-
    ten when they tell me about their problems; I don't offer to help.
I am often irritable with those around me, for example, I snap at people
    or criticise easily.
I show less affection.
I take part in fewer activities than I used to, for example, I go to fewer
    parties or social events.
I am cutting down the length of visits with friends.
I avoid having visitors.

My sexual activity is decreased.

I often express concern over what might be happening to my health.

I talk less with other people.

I make many demands on other people, for example, I insist that they do things for me or tell them how to do things.

I stay alone much of the time.

I am disagreeable with my family, for example, I act spitefully or stubbornly.

I frequently get angry with my family; for example, I hit them, scream or throw things at them.

I isolate myself as much as I can from the rest of my family.

I pay less attention to the children.

I refuse contact with my family; for example, I turn away from them.

I do not look after my children or family as well as I usually do.

I do not joke with members of my family as much as I usually do.

Emotions

I say how bad or useless I am, for example, that I am a burden on others.

I laugh or cry suddenly.

I often moan or groan because of pain or discomfort.

I have attempted suicide.

I behave nervously or restlessly.

I keep rubbing or holding areas of my body that hurt or are uncomfortable.

I am irritable and impatient with myself; for example, I run myself down, I swear at myself, I blame myself for things that happen.

I talk hopelessly about the future.

I get sudden frights.

Ambulation

I walk shorter distances or often stop for a rest.

I do not walk up or down hills.

I only use stairs with a physical aid, for example, a handrail, or stick or crutches.

I only go up and down stairs with assistance from someone else.

I get about in a wheelchair.

I do not walk at all.

I walk by myself but with some difficulty; for example, I limp, wobble, stumble or have a stiff leg.

I only walk with help from someone else.

I go up and down stairs more slowly, for example, one step at a time or I often have to stop.

I do not use stairs at all.

I get about only by using a walking frame, crutches, stick, walls or hold onto furniture.

I walk more slowly.

Eating

I eat much less than usual.

I feed myself but only with specially prepared food or special utensils.

I eat special or different food: for example, I follow a soft food, bland, low salt, low fat or low sugar diet.

I eat no food at all, but take liquids.

I just pick or nibble at my food.

I drink less fluids.

I feed myself with help from someone else.

I do not feed myself at all, but have to be fed.

Interviewer may code: I eat no food at all except by tubes or intravenous infusion.

Communication

I have trouble writing or typing.

I communicate mostly by nodding my head, pointing, or using sign language, or other gestures.

My speech is understood only by a few people who know me well.

I often lose control of my voice when I talk; for example, my voice gets louder or softer, or changes unexpectedly.

I don't write except to sign my name.

I carry on conversation only when very close to other people, or looking directly at them.

I speak with difficulty; for example, I get stuck for words, I stutter, I stammer, I slur my words.

I am understood with difficulty.

I do not speak clearly when I am under stress.

Work

Do you do work other then managing the home?

If "Yes", complete the work section, below.

If "No":

Are you retired?

If you are retired, was your retirement due to your health?

If you are not retired, but are not working, is this due to your health? *If "Yes", please tick the first item in this section, and skip the rest of the questions. If "No", please skip this section.*

I do not work at all (includes retired because of health).

I do part of my job at home.

I am not getting as much work done as usual.

I often get irritable with my workmates; for example, I snap at them or criticize them easily.

I work shorter hours.

I only do light work.

I only work for short periods of time, or often stop to rest.

I work at my usual job, but with some changes; for example, I use different tools or special aids, or I swap jobs with someone else.

I do not do my job as carefully or accurately as usual.

CHAPTER 9

Health status to quality
of life measurement

Danny A. Ruta and Andrew M. Garratt

Introduction

This chapter is in two parts. In the first part a "working" definition of
quality of life – the extent to which hopes and ambitions are matched by
experience – is proposed. This definition is comprehensive and gener-
alizable enough to be compatible with the diversity of perspectives and
theories expounded in the medical, behavioural and social science literature. Arriving at such a definition also requires us to draw upon two
important ideas developed in philosophy.

In the second part we examine two instruments which, when considered in the light of the definition proposed, are judged to be quality of
life measures. These are the Schedule for the Evaluation of Individual
Quality of Life (SEIQoL) (O' Boyle et al. 1992) and the Patient Generated
Index of Quality of Life (PGI) (Ruta et al. in press, a). Their relative merits
and disadvantages are discussed with respect to the desired measurement properties of validity, reliability, responsiveness and practicability.

What is "Quality of Life?"

A survey of the medical literature alone between 1989–93 under the
search term "Quality of Life" will generate around 1500 published
papers. The vast majority of these define quality of life, either explicitly
or implicitly, in terms of physical and mental functioning and wellbeing, focusing on what people can and cannot do. In the past, other

components such as financial security (McFarlane et al. 1981), life satisfaction (Neugarten et al. 1961), and mastery or control over one's life (Dupuy 1978, Guyatt et al. 1985) have also been included. In trying to arrive at a useful definition of quality of life very few researchers have appreciated the need to distinguish the factors necessary to sustain life, that enhance or impair the enjoyment of living, from whatever it is that we stay alive for. For most people, good health is not the end to which we aspire as human beings; it is simply the means to achieving an end, whatever that may be. To define what is a good (or bad) quality of life requires us to define exactly what it is that makes life worth living – its purpose. Seeking the answer to such a challenging question is certainly not the sole prerogative of health researchers. Many fields of art and science have addressed the same fundamental question of life's ultimate meaning and purpose – it is a common theme that unites them all. Indeed two key concepts – subjectivity and relativity – have characterized the Western twentieth century world-view regardless of disciplinary perspective. Together they provide the conceptual basis for a definition of quality of life.

The subjective (sometimes referred to as phenomenological) approach to the study of man takes as its starting point the experience of individuals; their subjective interpretation of events and the meaning they are able to find in them. It acknowledges that all phenomena are perceived through the distorting medium of the senses, and the meaning we ascribe to the world around us is a product of selective interpretation, itself influenced by personal attitudes and feelings. The notion of relativity grew out of the recognition, in the physical and social sciences, that many of the rules or laws which were thought to govern both the physical world and the actions of people in society, and which were considered to be universally valid, were only true in relation to a particular frame of reference. In a relativistic world, there is no unique or privileged vantage point from which it is possible to observe the "true" nature of physical events, or to make "correct" moral judgements.

A definition of quality of life

What then is the relevance of these two traditions for the development of quality of life measures in medical care? To begin with it is clear that any definition of quality of life must address the question of what it is that makes an individual's life worth living and gives it purpose. It is also clear that a definition will not be derived from any survey seeking to elicit answers to the question "what is a good quality of life (for you)?". Such surveys have been conducted, and inevitably they have produced an extensive list of different areas and activities of living (Dalkey et al. 1972, Age Concern 1974, Farquhar 1991), compelling us to acknowledge that the answer is "as varied as individual personalities" (Gough et al. 1983).

A subjectivist and relativistic philosophy maintains that we cannot specify that "X, Y and Z" make life worth living and give it purpose; one person's goal is seen as purposeless from another's standpoint. It also draws us irresistibly to another conclusion; that having a purpose is the purpose of life, and the extent to which individuals' goals are achieved determines how "good" or "bad" they perceive the quality of their life to be. If it is to have meaning and relevance, quality of life must be defined in individual terms. Calman (1984) defines quality of life as "the extent to which a person's hopes and ambitions are matched and fulfilled by experience". This definition not only meets the criteria of comprehensiveness and generalizability, but has already been adopted by many in the clinical research field (Cohen 1982, Presant 1984, Dupuis 1988). Calman, for example, has stated that to improve quality of life it is necessary to "narrow the gap between a person's hopes and expectations and what actually happens" (Calman 1984).

This definition of quality of life will not find favour with everyone. It has two very important, and at first glance paradoxical, implications which need to be carefully considered. First, if perceived quality of life is determined by the gap between a person's reality and their hopes and expectations, then a high perceived quality of life may stem from a low expectation. For example an elderly person who has learnt to live with an arthritic hip, and is ignorant of the improvement that might be possible as a result of surgery, may have a high perceived quality of life because their expectation is close to reality. Secondly, patients could have their perceived quality of life improved through a change or reduction in their expectations without any change in their reality. For example, a doctor may help an athlete with an irreversible paraplegia to come to terms with the limitations that this condition places on their life, and thus enable them to enjoy life, because their expectations have changed.

The problem with these scenarios stems from an inability to fully accept the subjectivist and relativistic view. Without them, one is drawn to form two value judgements; first, some hopes and expectations are genuine, while others are unreal. Secondly, it is unethical to improve quality of life by reducing expectations; conversely, it is ethical to raise awareness and thereby expectation, even if this results in unhappiness and discontentment. In a relativistic world, the distinction between real and unreal expectations is meaningless and irrelevant. Individuals' expectations are formed by their perception and interpretation of the world around them, which may lead them to be contented or miserable. The expectations that some call unreal are valid for the people that subscribe to them: they simply conflict with the expectations of others. The happiness that they experience because the gap between reality and expectation is narrow, is also valid for them. The patient who is experiencing excruciating leg pain caused by a trapped nerve, is no more incapacitated than the patient with equally excruciating non-organic, psychosomatic pain.

If one accepts the subjectivist/relativistic view that all expectations are valid, and also the earlier premise that quality of life is the end to which we aspire as individuals, then the second value judgement – that it is unethical to improve quality of life by reducing expectations – also becomes untenable. The doctor who counselled the young paraplegic and improved their perceived quality of life has not acted unethically; for a doctor intentionally to elevate a patient's expectation beyond his present experience without altering the reality of his daily life is to condemn him to a poorer quality of life.

Two measures of quality of life: the schedule for the evaluation of individual quality of life (SEIQoL) and the patient generated index (PGI)

If quality of life is defined as the gap between reality and expectations, then a measure of quality of life that can validly quantify this gap must be characterized by at least three of the following key properties. First, it must allow patients to specify those areas or activities which have relevance and meaning in the context of their daily lives, and which they consider to be of greatest importance. Secondly, it should allow patients to assess the extent to which reality matches expectation in each of their specified areas. Thirdly, it must incorporate individual patients' own valuations of the relative importance of their chosen areas. In addition, if an instrument is intended for use as an evaluative tool, it must give patients the opportunity to re-assess both the choice and the relative importance of their specified areas when changes in perceived quality of life are assessed over time. We are aware of only two measures reported in the literature which attempt to incorporate these key properties. They are: the Schedule for the Evaluation of Individual Quality of Life (SEIQoL) (McGee et al. 1991, O'Boyle et al. 1992, O'Boyle et al. 1993) and the Patient Generated Index (PGI) (Ruta et al. in press, a).

The SEIQoL

The SEIQoL was developed by O' Boyle and colleagues (McGee et al. 1991, O'Boyle et al. 1992), adapting a technique known as Judgement Analysis (JA) (Stewart 1988). The JA procedure uses multiple regression to model the various factors influencing a particular judgement or decision, and allows the relative importance of each to be quantified (Policy PC 1986). The SEIQoL takes the form of a semi-structured interview and may be administered both to patients and healthy members of the general population. It is completed in three stages. In the first stage, respondents are asked to list the five areas of life they judge to be most important in assessing overall quality of life. Respondents who find it difficult to list five areas are provided with a prompt list of eight possibilities (e.g. family, relationships). In the second stage, they are asked to rate each nominated area on a visual analogue scale from "As good as could possibly be" to "As bad as could possibly be". These ratings are then transferred by the respondent to a bar chart, each area represented by a separate bar (see Fig. 9.1). Respondents are then asked to rate their overall quality of life on a single visual analogue scale. In the third stage, respondents are presented with 30 hypothetical profiles randomly generated by computer. These are displayed as bar charts and are labelled with respondents' nominated areas. They are then asked to rate the overall quality of life score associated with each profile on a visual analogue scale. From these ratings, it is possible to estimate the relative weight attached to each nominated area using multiple regression analysis. Finally, an overall quality of life score for each individual is calculated by multiplying each nominated area by its corresponding weight and summing across the five areas to produce an index score between zero and 100.

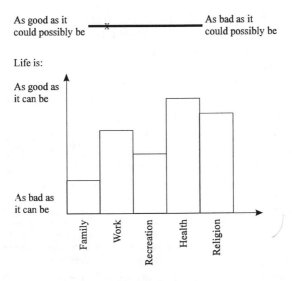

Figure 9.1 The SEIQOL: bar chart depicting current level of functioning on one individual's five nominated areas of life (Source: McGee et al. 1991).

The PGI

The PGI derives from a technique known as the priority evaluator method, developed by Hoinville (1977) to aid town planners to take account of the preferences of potential residents. The PGI was developed by Ruta and colleagues (in press, a) for use in routine clinical practice and was therefore designed as a self-completed questionnaire. Because of the nature of its design the PGI cannot be administered to healthy people – and therefore cannot be used to generate comparative norms. Like the SEIQOL, the PGI is completed in three stages (see Table 9.1). The first stage asks patients to list the five most important areas or activities of their life affected by their condition. The second stage asks patients to rate how badly affected they are in each of their chosen areas on a scale of zero to 100, where zero represents the worst they can imagine for themselves and 100 represents exactly as they would like to be. A sixth box is provided to enable them to rate all other areas of their life not previously mentioned. This may include areas of their life affected by their medical condition but not important enough to be included in the top five boxes as well as areas of their life which might be unrelated to their condition or even to their health. In the third stage, they are asked to imagine that they can improve some or all of the chosen areas of their life. They are "given" 60 "points" which they can choose to spend across one or more areas, reflecting the relative importance they attach to potential improvements in those areas. Finally by multiplying each of the six ratings by the proportion of points allocated to that area and summing, an index is generated between zero and 100. A copy of the PGI for use with patients with low back pain is reproduced at the end of this chapter.

Table 9.1 Stages in the completion of the PGI (Source: Ruta et al. 1993).

Stage I Area or activity	Stage II Score out of 100		Stage III Spend your points		Stage IV Total score
1. Work suffers	10	×	10/60	=	1.7
2. Makes me moody	30	×	10/60	=	5.0
3. Always thinking	30	×	5/60	=	2.5
4. Can't play with kids	50	×	20/60	=	16.7
5. My sex life suffers	70	×	10/60	=	11.7
6. All other aspects of your life not mentioned above	90	×	5/60	=	7.5
				Total =	45.0

A comparison of the SEIQoL with the PGI

The SEIQoL and the PGI are conceptually quite similar. Both instruments attempt to satisfy the requirements for a valid quality of life measure outlined above. They both allow patients to define quality of life in a way that has meaning for them, to assess the extent to which reality departs from their own expectations, and to value the relative importance of improvement in their chosen areas of life. However, there are important differences between the two methods. The SEIQoL asks patients to nominate the five most important areas of life, while the PGI asks for the most important areas of life affected by the medical condition, and two completely different techniques are used to elicit the relative weights for the chosen areas. Before an instrument can be recommended for use as an evaluative measure of quality of life, empirical evidence is required to establish its validity, reliability, responsiveness to change and practicability as a routine tool in quality of life assessment. The extent to which these criteria are met by each instrument will now be examined.

Instrument reliability

Reliability may be defined as the extent to which measurements on the same individual under different circumstances produce the same results (Streiner & Norman 1989). If an instrument is intended as an outcome measure, then it must demonstrate good test-retest reliability; i.e. observations on the same individuals separated by some interval of time must be similar (Streiner & Norman 1989). Streiner & Norman (1989) suggest that it is reasonable to demand test-retest reliability coefficients over 0.5 for group comparisons, although coefficients of 0.85 (Weiner & Stewart 1984)–0.94 (Kelly 1927) have been recommended when an instrument is to be used to make decisions concerning individuals.

The retest reliability of the SEIQoL has been assessed in a sample of 20 control subjects selected from a general practitioner list, as part of a prospective study of unilateral total hip replacement (O'Boyle et al. 1992). These controls were matched for age, sex and socio-economic status with 20 patients undergoing surgery. They completed the SEIQoL in their homes on two occasions 32 weeks apart. On the second occasion, subjects were provided with their original five chosen areas and asked to generate new ratings and weights. A test-retest reliability coefficient of 0.88 was achieved (O'Boyle et al. 1992).

PGI retest reliability has been assessed in a sample of 111 patients experiencing low back pain (Ruta et al. in press, a). A postal version of the PGI was mailed to patients on two occasions separated by a two week interval. The second questionnaire included a question asking patients if their health had improved, got worse, or remained the same since completing the first questionnaire. For patients reporting no change in health between the first and second set of responses, a test-retest reliability coefficient of 0.7 (p < 0.001) was achieved (Ruta et al. in press, a).

Both the SEIQoL and the PGI exceed the level of 0.5 required for group comparisons (Streiner & Norman 1989). The reliability coefficient of 0.88 obtained for the SEIQoL suggests that it may also be suitable for monitoring quality of life in individuals (Kelly 1927). This result is particularly impressive when one considers the 32 week interval between administrations. However in the SEIQoL study, subjects were provided with their previous chosen areas when completing their second interview, while in the PGI study, patients completed the retest questionnaire "blind" (with the result that patients made an average 1.7 changes in their choice of areas) (Ruta et al. in press, a). It is possible that a higher reliability coefficient could be obtained for the PGI if, as in the SEIQoL study, patients were provided with their previous responses when completing follow-up questionnaires. It has been suggested that this approach leads to an artificial improvement in reliability, with respondents repeating their previous response irrespective of any true change (Jacobsen 1965). If this were so, any improvement in reliability would be accompanied by a reduction in responsiveness to change. Guyatt found this not to be the case in his study of patients with chronic cardiorespiratory disease (Guyatt et al. 1985).

Criterion validity

Validity is the extent to which an instrument measures what is intended (Streiner & Norman 1989). The two approaches commonly used to test for validity are criterion and construct validity. Criterion validity assesses the extent to which a new measure is correlated with existing measures of the concept under study, sometimes referred to as "gold standard" measures because their validity has been clearly established. If the new measure and a gold standard are administered simultaneously, and a high correlation is demonstrated, then the new measure is considered to possess "concurrent" criterion validity. If a gold standard is administered at some time in the future, but its results can be predicted by the new measure, then the new measure demonstrates "predictive" criterion validity. The problem in quality of life research is that no gold standard exists. One solution to this problem is to correlate a new instrument which purports to measure quality of life with a gold standard measure of a concept that is closely related to quality of life – such as health status. If good health is important in achieving a high perceived quality of life, and conversely if poor health prevents the enjoyment of work, family life and other activities, then we would expect a valid quality of life measure to show a moderate correlation with measures of health and disease – especially when administered to a group of people suffering ill health. If the correlation were too high – i.e. greater than 0.8 – this would imply that the new instrument is measuring health status rather than quality of life, while a very weak correlation – i.e. less than 0.2 – would suggest that the measure was invalid.

In the SEIQOL hip replacement study (O'Boyle et al. 1992), patients' health status was assessed using a general measure of health – the McMaster Health Index Questionnaire (MHIQ) – and a condition-specific measure of disease – the Arthritis Impact Measurement Scale (AIMS). The MHIQ is a 59-item questionnaire designed to measure physical, social and emotional functioning (Chambers et al. 1976). Responses to items on these three dimensions are summed to produce a single index score. The AIMS comprises nine scales measuring different aspects of health (Meenan et al. 1980) (e.g. mobility, dexterity, pain). As with the MHIQ, an overall score may be generated by summing across the scales. Both measures have been subjected to extensive tests of reliability and validity (Chambers et al. 1982, 1984, Chambers et al. 1987, Meenan et al. 1980, 1982, 1984, Brown et al. 1984). When SEIQOL scores were compared with those from the MHIQ and the AIMS, correlation coefficients of 0.21 and 0.25 respectively, were achieved.

In the PGI study of low back pain, health status was also assessed with a combination of general and disease-specific measures. General health was measured by the Short-Form 36-item Health Survey Questionnaire. The SF-36 is designed to measure health across three dimensions using eight separate scales (Ware & Sherbourne 1992) (e.g. physical functioning, mental health, pain), and has been validated in the United States (McHorney et al. 1992, McHorney et al. 1993) and in the UK (Brazier et al. 1992, Garratt et al. 1993b, Jenkinson et al. 1993a). The severity of low back pain was assessed by the Aberdeen Low Back Pain Scale (Ruta et al. in press, b), a 19-item questionnaire devised from questions commonly used in the clinical assessment of patients presenting with low back pain. Patients' scores on the PGI demonstrated significant correlations with all eight SF-36 scales (see Table 9.2). Correlation coefficients ranged from 0.13 (with general health perceptions) to 0.47 (with pain). A correlation coefficient of 0.42 was achieved with the low back pain scale.

Table 9.2   Criterion validity between PGI score, the clinical (low back pain) score and the eight dimensions of the SF-36 health profile (Source: Ruta et al. 1993).

Measure	Correlation with the PGI score
A *Low back pain clinical score*	0.42**
B *SF-36 health profile scores:*	
Physical functioning	0.26**
Social functioning	0.38**
Role limitations attributed to physical problems	0.27**
Role limitations attributed to emotional problems	0.18**
Mental health	0.29**
Energy/fatigue	0.27**
Pain	0.47**
General health perception	0.13*

** Significant at the 0.1% level
* Significant at the 1% level

For both the SEIQOL and PGI, the degree of correlation with established health status measures reported in these studies lends support to claims made by the instruments' authors that they assess quality of life. The PGI, however, appears to magnify the effect of impaired health status on quality of life. This is reflected in the moderately high correlations observed with certain SF-36 scales and with the clinically derived measure of disease severity. This apparent "bias" towards health is probably the result of a "framing effect". The PGI asks patients first to nominate the five most important areas of their life affected by their medical condition, focusing their attention on health. In order to generate a true quality of life index, patients are then given the opportunity to include all other aspects of life, but this potentially large and varied group of areas and activities is relegated to a single box in the subsequent scoring/weighting procedures. The SEIQOL does not manifest this kind of framing effect, and may therefore be a more valid measure of overall quality of life. The PGI, on the other hand, may be more sensitive to the effects of treatment, and therefore more appropriate for use in clinical evaluations (see *Responsiveness to change* below).

Construct validity

Construct validity assesses the extent to which a new measure is related to criteria derived from an established clinical or social theory or "construct" (Streiner & Norman 1989). One might hypothesize for example, that quality of life is related to socio-economic status, with the least deprived enjoying the highest quality of life. If individuals' scores on a new measure are shown to relate to their socio-economic status as predicted by the theory, then the instrument is said to demonstrate "convergent" construct validity (Streiner & Norman 1989). Conversely, one might hypothesize that quality of life was independent of age. If the new measure is shown to be uncorrelated with age, then it is said to possess "discriminant" construct validity (Streiner & Norman 1989). This approach to validity testing does not require the existence of an established gold standard. However a test of construct validity is only as "good" as the underlying hypothesis on which it is based. In practice it is often difficult to decide whether an observed lack of convergent validity is due to an invalid measure or a poorly constructed theory.

The developers of the SEIQoL have assessed construct validity by focusing on the various methods employed to derive a SEIQoL quality of life score, rather than testing the validity of the final score itself (O'Boyle et al. 1992, O'Boyle et al. 1993). From data provided by the SEIQoL hip replacement study, for example, the following hypotheses were tested: respondents completing the SEIQoL nominate areas or activities of life that are not elicited by conventional measures, SEIQoL scores using predetermined areas or activities of life derived from traditional health status measures are less sensitive to improvement in quality of life following surgery compared with SEIQoL scores using areas elicited by patients, individuals vary considerably in the relative importance they attach to the five areas as reflected in the weights they assign to each, and for a given individual the relative importance of each area may change over time.

Table 9.3. shows the frequency of different areas or activities of life mentioned by patients and controls in the hip replacement study. Although the most frequently mentioned areas – social/leisure activities, family, and personal health – will be found in most conventional health status questionnaires, certain areas elicited by the SEIQoL – e.g. religion, finances, family health – would not normally be included. When patients undergoing hip replacement completed the SEIQoL using five pre-determined areas of life – physical functioning, social functioning, emotional functioning, living conditions and general health – derived from conventional questionnaires, a non-significant improvement in quality of life score was detected (4.5 points) at 7.5 months postoperatively (O'Boyle et al. 1993). When SEIQOL scores were generated using patients' own elicited areas of life, a statistically significant improvement was detected (9.1 points p < 0.02) (O'Boyle et al. 1992). Considerable variation was found between individuals in the weights assigned to different areas of life when respondents were asked to complete the SEIQOL using the five pre-determined areas (O'Boyle et al. 1993). There was also evidence that patients changed the relative importance attached to certain areas over time. Patients who underwent hip replacement assigned a mean weight of 0.28 to general health pre-operatively; at 7.5 months post-operatively this had increased to 0.35 (O'Boyle et al. 1993).

Table 9.3 Patients nominating various areas of life as essential to their overall quality of life (Source: O'Boyle et al. 1992).

	Controls		Patients	
	n	%	n	%
Social/leisure activities	18	(90)	15	(75)
Family	18	(90)	14	(70)
Personal health	14	(70)	10	(50)
Relationships	10	(50)	9	(45)
Religion	9	(45)	9	(45)
Work	8	(40)	8	(45)
Finances	6	(30)	10	(50)
Family health	5	(25)	1	(5)
Independence	5	(25)	10	(50)
Living conditions	4	(20)	3	(15)
Miscellaneous	2	(10)	3	(15)
Intellectual function	1	(5)	2	(1)
Happiness*	0	(0)	0	(0)

* $p < 0.05$ for McNemar comparisons between groups; all other comparisons not significant.

In the PGI study of low back pain, construct validity was assessed by relating the total PGI score to a number of criteria derived from clinical and social theory (Ruta et al. in press, a). The following hypotheses were tested: non-referred patients have higher PGI scores than referred patients, patients taking analgesics have lower scores than patients not taking analgesics, scores are related to symptom severity as perceived by the GP, positively correlated with home ownership, higher in married than in single patients and lower in unemployed than in employed patients.

Table 9.4. shows that referred patients have a statistically significant lower mean PGI score than patients being managed in general practice. Scores were also related to the use and strength of analgesics, and to symptom severity as assessed by the GP. Patients who owned their own homes had higher mean scores than those living in rented accommodation. Married patients and those in employment had higher scores than single and unemployed patients respectively.

Table 9.4 Validity: PGI score by referral, severity, medication, housing tenure, marital status and employment (Source: Ruta et al. 1993).

Variable	Number of patients	PGI score
Referred to hospital		
No	206	34.7*
Yes	153	29.2
GP severity rating		
None	6	44.7
Mild	81	37.0
Moderate	105	32.5
Severe	12	36.0
Analgesics being taken:		
No	64	36.9
Yes	295	31.6
Analgesic strength:		
Mild–moderate	58	36.1
Moderate–severe	172	33.1
Housing tenure:		
Privately owned	255	33.4
Rented	104	29.7
Marital status:		
Married	278	32.6
Single	78	31.4
Employment status:		
Part or full time	234	33.4
Unemployed	8	28.0

The approach used by O'Boyle and colleagues to assess the SEIQoL does not strictly address the issue of construct validity. Good evidence is provided for the validity of the SEIQoL technique as a means of eliciting the most important areas of life, however this is not the same as demonstrating that the SEIQoL is measuring what is intended, i.e. perceived quality of life. A more appropriate approach to validity testing has been adopted with the PGI. An attempt is made to demonstrate that the total PGI score is related to specified variables in accordance with an established theory or "hypothetical construct". However, interpretation of the results is difficult and ambiguous. PGI scores appear to be related to differences in disease severity as assessed by the GP, analgesic use, employment, marital status and home ownership in a manner predicted by clinical and social theory, but differences in the scores are small and nonsignificant. Do these findings indicate that the PGI has poor convergent validity, or do they indicate the weakness of the underlying theory? An alternative hypothesis might postulate that individuals adapt their expectations to suit their particular social or economic circumstances. In this case the observed lack of differences in PGI scores with regard to employment, marital status and home ownership could be construed as evidence of discriminant construct validity.

Responsiveness to change

If a quality of life measure is to be used to evaluate the outcome of care for patients, then it must be shown to be responsive, or sensitive, to clinically significant change in quality of life over time. Several different methods have been proposed to evaluate the magnitude of change in a way that allows meaningful comparisons to be made between instruments (Guyatt et al. 1987, Kazis et al. 1989, Liang et al. 1990). Kazis and colleagues (1989) have argued for the use of the "effect size" as a simple standardized index of responsiveness to change. In order to calculate the effect size for a quality of life measure, the mean difference between quality of life scores at two points in time is divided by the standard deviation of the scores at baseline. An effect size of around 0.2 indicates a small effect or clinical change, 0.5 moderate and 0.8 or greater a large effect (Kazis et al. 1989).

In the SEIQoL hip replacement study, quality of life was measured in 20 patients during routine pre-surgical assessment six weeks prior to surgery, and again 26 weeks post-operatively. In the PGI low back pain study, 136 patients were assessed within two weeks of consulting their general practitioner, and again after one year. The mean change in scores, standard deviations and effect sizes are shown in Table 9.5. Effect sizes of 0.48 and 0.61 were seen with the SEIQoL and PGI respectively.

Table 9.5 Responsiveness to change: mean scores, standard deviations, and effect sizes for patients undergoing hip replacement (SEIQoL) and patients with low back pain (PGI).

	Mean score (SD) Before	Mean score (SD) After	Effect size
[1]SEIQoL	61.6	70.7*	0.48
Hip replacement study	(18.8)	(11.2)	
[2]PGI	30.6	41.1**	0.61
Low back pain study	(17.1)	(20.3)	

* Mean scores of 20 patients 7.5 months after hip replacement
** Mean scores of 136 patients with low back pain one year after consulting their GP
Sources: [1]O'Boyle et al. 1993. [2]Ruta et al. unpublished data

The magnitude of an effect size for a particular measure is determined by several factors other than instrument responsiveness. The variability in the population being studied with regard to socio-demographic characteristics, disease type and severity, the presence of other co-morbid conditions and the size of the true clinical effect will all have an influence. An ideal comparison of the responsiveness of two measures would administer both instruments to a single patient sample in which all patients were receiving an identical treatment of known clinical effectiveness. A degree of caution should be exercised in interpreting effect sizes reported for the SEIQoL and PGI from two very different studies. In both studies, the two measures were able to detect a moderate clinical change over time. However, a considerable mean improvement in quality of life would be expected from hip replacement (Williams 1985, Liang et al. 1986, Frankel et al. 1991), while few treatments for low back pain have been shown to be of clear value (Quebec Task Force 1987). The fact that a larger effect size was seen with the PGI than with the SEIQoL provides some empirical evidence that, because of its focus on health, the PGI may be more sensitive to the effects of treatment.

Practicability

An instrument intended for use as an outcome measure should satisfy fairly stringent criteria of validity, reliability and responsiveness. However, these criteria "cannot and should not be applied to the exclusion of more practical considerations" (Wilkin et al. 1992, 1993). Indeed many of the newer health status measures have been developed specifically with these practical considerations in mind, often sacrificing some degree of reliability and validity for greater simplicity, compliance and ease of administration (McHorney et al. 1992). When assessing the practicability of a new measure, the particular clinical setting in which the developers intend it to be used should always be borne in mind.

Potential applications of the SEIQoL are not explicitly identified by the instrument's authors, but as the name implies, it seems to have been designed primarily as an evaluation tool for use in clinical trials. In this context, it is applicable in most clinical situations (the authors caution against its use in young children and patients suffering from impaired cognitive function or severe depression). Completion rates in five reported studies ranged from 87% to 100% (O'Boyle et al. 1993). Few problems were encountered when the SEIQoL was administered to the elderly; a normative study of quality of life in the healthy aged with a mean age of 73.7 years achieved a completion rate of 90.4% (O'Boyle et al. 1993). Because it can be administered to healthy individuals, normative values can be derived for comparative purposes (O'Boyle et al. 1992). The fact that it is interviewer-administered, however, and the 30 minutes required to complete the judgement analysis (although a direct weighting procedure is being developed which takes about 3 minutes – O'Boyle, unpublished data), precludes its use as a routine measure of outcome in busy clinical settings.

The PGI can also be administered by an interviewer. In this format, we have found the completion rate approaches 100%. The major practical advantage of the PGI over the SEIQoL, however, is in its use as a self-administered postal questionnaire, which considerably widens its potential application. Problems of responder bias have been encountered with the postal PGI. In the low back pain study for example, 37% of respondents returning a questionnaire failed to complete the PGI correctly (Ruta et al. in press, a). These patients were found to be significantly older and less well-educated than those completing it correctly. Unlike the SEIQoL, normative values cannot be derived for the PGI, because it is condition specific.

Conclusion

Both instruments are sufficiently reliable for group comparisons. The SEIQOL appears suitable for monitoring quality of life in individuals, and it is possible that the PGI could also achieve this level of reliability if patients are provided with their previous chosen areas when completing follow-up questionnaires. In the absence of a gold standard, both instruments were assessed for criterion validity by comparison with disease-specific and generic measures of health status. The SEIQOL and PGI both achieve correlation coefficients consistent with a quality of life measure – i.e. not too high and not too low. The higher correlations observed for the PGI suggest that it may magnify the effect of impaired health on perceived quality of life.

In testing for construct validity, the SEIQOL has been shown to elicit important areas of life in an individualized manner, but no evidence is provided for the validity of the quality of life score that it generates. Although more appropriate tests of construct validity were conducted for the PGI, the results are difficult to interpret. There is good evidence of responsiveness to clinical change for both instruments, and some evidence that, because of its focus on health, the PGI may be more sensitive to the effects of treatment. In terms of practicability, the SEIQOL is largely restricted to use in evaluation studies. It does have a clear advantage over the PGI, however, in that normative data on perceived quality of life can be obtained from healthy populations. The PGI has potential for wider application as a complementary tool in routine outcomes assessment, although in order to reduce responder bias, more work is required to develop a more concise and simplified postal version.

In conclusion, the SEIQOL and the PGI attempt to measure the gap between peoples' hopes and expectations and reality in a way which has meaning and relevance in the context of their daily lives. Both measures require further evaluation, and future research may focus on developing instruments which combine elements of each, but together they offer an exciting new approach to the problem of measuring quality of life.

The Patient Generated Index

The PGI is constantly undergoing development and improvement, and the copy of the schedule reproduced below is for reference only.

Potential users should contact either: Dr Danny Ruta, Department of Public Health Medicine, Tayside Health Board, Vernonholme, Riverside Drive, Dundee or Mr Andrew Garratt, Department of Public Health, University of Aberdeen, Foresterhill, Aberdeen, for information on the most appropriate and up-to-date version available.

The PGI can be used to assess quality of life in any illness. The example reproduced below is for the assessment of low back pain.

How you are affected

This questionnaire is in three stages. When you are filling in each stage, we would like you to think about when you were at your worst with your back pain in the last month. If you are at your worst now, then think about how you feel now.

Stage one
At this stage, we would like you to think of the different areas in your life, or activities in your life that have been affected by your *back pain* in the last month. When you think of areas or activities, you might think of some small area or activity which may be quite personal and special to you like "I can't play with my kids".

We would like you to write the *five* most important areas or activities of your life that are affected by your back pain in the boxes provided in the *Stage 1* boxes below. Put one area or activity in each box.

You may be able to think of more than five areas but you can only write down the five most important ones. *Note:* The PGI may be administered to respondents with a list of items to act as "triggers" for those who cannot think of areas influenced by their illness. Such items are generated from in-depth interviews, previous responses to the questionnaire etc.

You don't have to write down five areas of your life if you don't feel that five areas of your life have been affected. If you have less than five, you can write "none" in the empty boxes and move on to stage two.

If you feel that your life is not affected by your illness *at all*, then just send back the questionnaire with "none" in each box. In this case you don't need to go on to stages two and three.

Once you have written down the most important areas or activities that have been affected by your back pain, you can move on to stage two.

Stage two
Underneath the boxes you have completed, you will see a scale going from 0–100 in multiples of 10. This scale is supposed to show you how badly affected you are for each of the areas or activities you have mentioned. A score of zero would mean that when you were at your worst in the last month, you felt that this was really the worst you could imagine for yourself. The score of 100 is meant to represent exactly how you would like to be, in that area or activity of your life (even if it is impossible for you to reach).

For each area or activity that you have mentioned, write down a score out of 100 that you would give to reflect how you were affected when you were at your worst in the last month.

You will notice that we have filled in "all other aspects of your life" the final "area or activity". This is meant to include all the other areas of your life affected by your illness, but which are not important enough to go in the top five boxes. It will also include areas in your life which might be totally unaffected, like the size of your house.

You might suffer from another illness as well as your back pain, and any other areas that are affected by this illness would be included in this box.

Please give a score out of 100 to the "All other areas of your life" box the same way that you scored the other "areas and activities". Even if you leave the other boxes empty you must fill in this box.

Stage three
For the final stage, we would like you to imagine that we can grant you a wish to improve *any* area of your life, including the areas that have nothing to do with your back pain.

Imagine that you are given *60 points* to improve your score in any of the areas you have mentioned. You cannot have more than 60 points in total but you can spend them anyway you like. For example, you could give 10 points to each area or you might give 60 points to one area. The choice is yours to split the points up any way you like, but you cannot have more than 60 points in total.

If you don't give any points to an area in your life, you must try to imagine that this area will stay exactly as it is.

Go through the boxes in stage three and distribute your points to those areas or activities in which you would most like to improve. You can keep changing your mind until you feel that you have reached the best distribution of points. Remember that the total across all areas has to add up to 60.

Stage 1
area/activity
(e.g. sport)

Stage 2
score each area/
activity out of 100

Stage 3
spend your
60 points between
the different areas

Total number of points should add up to 60

All other aspects of your life not mentioned above

You must fill in this box

100 Exactly as you would like to be
 90 Close to how you would like to be
 80 Very good but not how you would like to be
 70 Good but not how you would like to be
 60 Between fair and good
 50 Fair
 40 Between poor and fair
 30 Poor but not the worst you could imagine
 20 Very poor but not the worst you could imagine
 10 Close to the worst you could imagine
  0 The worst you could imagine

You have finished this section. It will tell us how your back pain has affected your life and also which aspects of your life you would most like to see improved.

Reproduced by permission. © Danny Ruta, Andrew Garratt and Ian Russell.

CHAPTER 10

Subjective health assessment and distributive justice

Matthew G. Clayton and Andrew D. Williams

Introduction

This chapter explores, from the perspective of contemporary political philosophy, some of the possible benefits of patient subjective health assessment. It examines what information, if any, such assessment might provide which could facilitate improved medical decision-making. More specifically, it asks in what ways standard fixed format questionnaires can inform judgements concerning the just distribution of scarce public medical resources, taking as an example an increasingly popular instrument, the SF-36 Health Survey Questionnaire. In addressing this question, it disregards many other conceivable benefits. Some, for instance, might accrue to patients who are made more confident by the very act of attempting to acquire information from them even if, unbeknown to them, the information acquired was subsequently ignored. Others might accrue to private medical institutions, seeking for commercial reasons to ascertain clients' satisfaction with the service they have purchased. These benefits, however, are not our concern.

A second limit to the enquiry should also be noted at the outset. In making distributive decisions subjective health assessment might be relevant to establishing both the *probability of success* and the *moral urgency* of treating different individuals. In the former case, subjective health scores might, to some extent, indicate how effective a particular treatment would be for a specific patient. For example, perhaps treatment is more effective if patients are hopeful rather than depressed, and certain variables provide information about such facts. In the latter case, subjective health scores might support interpersonal comparative judgements about health status, both before and after treatment. Such judgements concern the extent of ill health experienced by any given individual, and to what extent such individuals benefit from medical care. They are relevant, in ways to be explained, to establishing the strength of those individuals' competing claims to scarce medical resources.

The chapter disregards the former and deals only with the second of these two considerations. It will be argued that the conception of health status implicit in the SF-36 incorporates two distinct kinds of concern. The former is attached to individuals' *capabilities*, that is, the types of action they can perform and types of physical and mental condition they can attain. The latter relates to their *welfare*, or the degree to which they take pleasure in, or are satisfied by their health, and their lives in general. The view is defended that while the nature of people's capabilities has moral relevance for distributive decisions involving scarce health care resources, there are serious moral objections to basing such decisions upon facts about people's welfare. Thus, subjective health assessment improves decision-making to the extent that it provides reliable information about patients' capabilities. The information it provides about their level of subjective contentment, however, is not of fundamental moral importance, although it may, as noted, be relevant to the prospects of successful treatment.

Distributive justice

Many agree that the primary purpose of public health care is to benefit individuals, by alleviating the burden of ill health. Fewer agree, however, exactly how the competing claims of distinct individuals for medical treatment are to be balanced. Indeed one of the central and perennial debates within political philosophy concerns distributive justice, or how, given scarce means, benefits and burdens should be divided between distinct individuals. In the case of securing a just distribution of public health care, this chapter will assume, without further argument, that there are at least two relevant concerns. First, it is relevant to ask to what extent a patient's health can be improved by treatment. Other things being equal, it is better to allocate a given quantity of medical resources to patients for whom they would do the most good. Thus, resources should be devoted to patients whose health would be improved to the greatest extent. Secondly, a morally adequate distribution of medical care must be sensitive to the seriousness of patients' medical needs. The more ill the patient is, the more urgent it is that curative medical care is provided. Other things being equal, the claims of the least healthy should have priority in the distribution of medical resources.

Difficult moral problems arise when these two considerations conflict. Suppose there are two patients, Ann who has chronic obstructive pulmonary disease, and Bob who has psoriasis. Ann's condition is worse than Bob's, but with the available medical resources physicians can improve Bob's health more than they can improve Ann's. Alternative moral theories prescribe different distributive policies in this context. Two extreme policies are (a) to maximize the amount of good health in society, which gives absolute priority to those whose health can be improved most, irrespective of how badly off they are, and (b) to maximize the health of the least healthy, which gives absolute priority to improving the condition of the least healthy in society, irrespective of the extent to which their health can be improved. A moderate view attaches moral weight to both considerations. It claims that it is more urgent to cure less healthy individuals but that in some cases a larger improvement in health of someone who is relatively healthier would be sufficient to override the concern for the least healthy in society. This position lacks the simplicity of the two extreme views but it has more intuitive plausibility. Since it disregards the numbers of individuals affected by a decision it may also be excessively simple, but this consideration is not relevant for present purposes.

Interpersonal comparison

The previous observations are significant for the following reason. If a health status scale is to facilitate improved decision-making about the allocation of scarce medical resources, then it must address the two aspects of distributive justice previously described. To do so, it must indicate how ill is a given individual, and enable physicians to ascertain how much better off she would become if a particular treatment were successful. Thus, a health measurement scale must be capable of identifying, at least roughly, the level of one person's health at various points in time, and the relative health of different persons. These requirements can be designated the *formal* conditions of moral adequacy for a questionnaire capable of measuring health status.

Perhaps, however, the most important conditions of moral adequacy of such scales are not formal but *substantive*. They concern questions such as the following. In what does ill health consist? What benefits should public medical care aim to provide? In addressing these questions the chapter turns to a parallel discussion within contemporary political philosophy of the notion of *advantage*.

Within political philosophy, and economics, a variety of criteria have been proposed as the standard of interpersonal comparison appropriate for examining the justice of basic social institutions (Cohen 1989, Scanlon 1991, 1993). Three of the most prominent standards construe an individual's level of advantage in terms of *access to economic resources*, *welfare*, and *capabilities* respectively (Dworkin 1981a, 1981b, Sen 1982). Below, the chapter will argue that the Short-Form 36 health survey questionnaire (SF-36), the development and validation of which has been discussed elsewhere in this text, presupposes that both welfare and capabilities are relevant criteria by which health status is defined. Prior to elucidating and evaluating these criteria, it is instructive to consider how both respond to deficiencies in access to economic resources as a possible construal of advantage.

It is sometimes argued that a just society would adopt access to economic resources as its standard of interpersonal comparison, and, thus, would ensure that everyone has their fair share of, for example, wealth and income (Rawls 1982). An attractive feature of this standard is that resources are flexible. They can be employed in the pursuit of many different life-plans. For example, lives of religious devotion and sporting competition both require resources if they are to be effectively pursued. Nevertheless, whilst economic resources are flexible with respect to differences in life-plans, they lack flexibility or sensitivity in a distinct, but no less relevant, dimension. Comparing individuals' levels of advantage only in terms of their access to economic resources is insensitive to differences between individuals in terms of their ability to use such resources (Arrow 1973, Sen 1990). It is unfair to give equal shares to a paraplegic and a fully able-bodied person, because the former requires more resources to attain the same goals.

This insensitivity is often diagnosed by describing the resource standard as *fetishistic*, since it misidentifies what is of ultimate importance in assessing advantage. It mistakenly treats economic resources as being fundamentally important, whereas in fact their value lies in them being one means, among others, for individuals to be able to attain certain states. There may be ways of trying to determine fair shares of economic resources in a way which is sensitive to morally relevant differences between persons. Nevertheless, the first stage in such a revision is to arrive at a plausible conception of individual advantage.

Appeals to welfare and to capabilities are distinct attempts to characterize a non-fetishistic standard of interpersonal comparison. Both agree that distributive decision-makers, when evaluating the contribution of economic, or medical, resources to individual advantage, should take into account the impact of such resources upon individuals' lives. They differ, however, in their view of which aspects of our lives are of ultimate importance for distributive justice. The welfarist claims that individual experience or preference satisfaction alone has value. Hence, an individual's level of advantage depends upon the extent to which her experience is pleasurable rather than painful, or her preferences are satisfied rather than frustrated. Opposing welfarism, Amartya Sen has suggested that interpersonal comparison should concern individuals' capability to perform, or attain, certain types of *function* (Sen 1982, 1992). Such functions include both specific types of action, such as walking, and specific non-intentional states, such as being well-nourished.

Whereas welfarist measures provide a subjectivist interpretation of advantage, the capability view provides a non-subjectivist interpretation in the following sense. A criterion is *subjectivist* if, and only if, it claims that advantage consists only in certain facts about people's mental states. Such facts, for example, might include the extent to which their experiences are pleasurable, or their preferences satisfied. In contrast, *non-subjectivist* criteria differ in at least two respects. First, they are broader insofar as they treat a wider range of facts as constituents of advantage. They claim that advantage at least partly consists in facts about individuals' lives which make reference to non-mental states. Such states could include, for example, their physical mobility or level of nutritional well-being. Secondly, they are narrower, insofar as they reject particular aspects of mental life, such as individuals' level of pleasure or desire-fulfilment, as aspects of advantage. They may, however, count as components of advantage some mental states, such as the existence of physical pain. Indeed a failure to do so would clearly be counter-intuitive. Welfare as such, however, is disregarded by non-subjectivist accounts of advantage such as capability standards. Before going on to explore the reasons for such exclusion, the chapter turns to examine the SF-36 health survey questionnaire.

The SF-36 health survey questionnaire

In discussing subjective health assessment it is important to note an important distinction between two respects in which an assessment may be subjective, which relates to the previous distinction between subjectivist and non-subjectivist accounts of advantage. A health status measure might involve a *subjective mode of assessment*. Such is the case if it relies on patients' beliefs about their own condition, such as their reports concerning their ability to breathe freely, see, hear, walk adequately etc. In so doing it may treat such capabilities as constitutive of health status, and regard patients' beliefs about them as reliable evidence about health status. It is subjective only in an unobjectionable evidential sense. It is not committed to a subjectivist account of advantage in the sense previously described, since it does not conceive of health as consisting in particular experiences or in preference-satisfaction. In contrast, a health status measure might concern a *subjective object of assessment*. It does if it treats patients' level of happiness or preference-satisfaction as at least partly constitutive of their health status. Thus, Ann enjoys a lower health status than Bob if she takes less pleasure from, or satisfaction in, her life.

As illustration consider the SF-36. It provides a method of health assessment that is subjective in both its mode and object. Many of its questions ask for patients' reports of their capability levels, and whether they have improved over time. For example, it enquires about limitations in physical activities such as walking, running, lifting, climbing, etc., and about occurrence of bodily pain. These questions appear to presuppose that health is defined, at least in part, in terms of capabilities, and that patients' reports are a reliable guide to such considerations. Nevertheless, certain aspects of the questionnaire regard health status in terms of one's satisfaction with one's life. For example, it asks whether over the past month one has felt: full of life, down in the dumps, calm and peaceful, downhearted and low, or happy. These are welfarist considerations.

A natural interpretation of the SF-36 is that it conceives health in terms of both capability and welfare. If this is correct, the usefulness of the questionnaire in making distributive decisions is dependent upon the resolution of possible conflicts between the two concerns. Take the case of Tiny Tim and Scrooge (Dworkin 1981a). In virtue of his physical disabilities Tiny Tim scores lower than Scrooge in terms of capability. Nevertheless, despite these disabilities, he is happier than Scrooge. If health status depends only upon welfare level, then social resources should be allocated to Scrooge rather than Tiny Tim. (This may involve the conversion of resources for medical care into non-medical resources.) However, if health status is exhaustively characterized by capability, then resources should be allocated to Tiny Tim to cure his disabilities or, if this is not possible, to seek to mitigate their effects through, for example, the use of a wheelchair.

How are these cases of conflict to be resolved? One strategy is to attach appropriate weights to the concerns for people's welfare and capability respectively. This is a difficult task, which in all likelihood could be done only roughly. If both are constituents of health, then one must know the degree to which each component matters. It is unclear how we should arrive at these judgements. In addition, even if one discovered the extent to which patients' happiness matters, there seem to be many epistemic and interpretative difficulties in measuring the relative happiness of different individuals. An alternative response to conflict between considerations of welfare and capability, which this chapter will pursue, is to disregard the welfarist component of health assessment questionnaires when making distributive decisions. Doing so overcomes some of the practical problems of identifying happiness, and the difficulty in weighing its relative importance in a non-arbitrary manner. Nevertheless, the reasons for eliminating welfare considerations are not merely practical but also ethical. There are serious principled objections to regarding welfare as constitutive of advantage and, thus, of health status. Insofar as the SF-36 does so, it is questionable.

Two problems for welfarism

Malformed preferences

In assessing their welfare the SF-36 seeks information about individuals' actual happiness. It asks, for example, whether one feels happy, full of

life, calm and peaceful, or down in the dumps. However, it is highly con-
testable that these qualities should be taken as constitutive of health status. The aspirations and preferences by which our welfare is determined
are sometimes shaped in circumstances which encourage an attitude of
resignation. Compare Challenged who is encouraged to adopt and pursue ambitious goals, with Checked, who through familial and peer pressure becomes satisfied with a life of few challenges. A problem for
welfarism is evident. Since the welfarist questions of subjective health
assessment relate to people's actual levels of satisfaction, they might
suggest that the welfare of Challenged and Checked are the same. However, as the example shows, one's actual welfare is an unreliable guide to
one's level of advantage. Checked, whose development has taken place
against an unpropitious background, is satisfied with having fewer
opportunities than others. Nevertheless, it is surely objectionable to treat
this satisfaction as indicative of her level of advantage when this is an
effect of deprivation. If, for example, Checked has been manipulated by
others, such that she is now satisfied with less in life, then it seems relevant to consider such facts in assessing her advantage. However, the
SF-36 ignores these important historical facts.

Attitudes of resignation may also be due to factors other than manipu-
lation, for which no individual is responsible. Consider the fable of *sour
grapes* (Elster 1982), in which the fox is unable to obtain the grapes.
Despite this inability the fox suffers no welfare loss for not having them
since he does not desire them because he believes them to be sour. However, his beliefs and desires are in part caused by the fact that the grapes
are unavailable to him. The problem of sour grapes, or *adaptive preference
formation*, is that there is a positive causal relationship between the quality or number of options which are available to a person and the quality
or number of preferences which she forms. Similar cases arise in medical
contexts. People may become resigned to their lack of capability and,
consequently, their actual welfare may be relatively high. It seems objectionable to judge their health status by reference to these malformed
preferences. Thus, either information about welfare should be disregarded in assessing health status, or it must be supplemented by other
considerations which qualify the extent to which actual welfare is a constituent of health.

There are at least two distinct conclusions about the rôle of welfare
within subjective health assessment which might be drawn from the previous line of reasoning. The first sweeping conclusion is that, because of

its dependence upon background conditions, welfare in any form is not a component of health status. However, a more modest conclusion is also available. It might instead be concluded that only some, but not all, considerations about welfare have been discredited. If a view of healthy preference formation can be articulated, then it may still be possible to regard some welfare information as morally relevant. For example, Richard Arneson suggests that in assessing advantage we should consider the level of satisfaction of one's ideally considered preferences, namely those preferences which a person would have, were she to deliberate rationally with full information (Arneson 1990: 163). Questions concerning welfare might then guide distributive decisions providing it could be ascertained that respondents were not reporting malformed preferences.

In this paper we do not endorse the first ambitious objection to subjective health assessment. Consideration of individuals' welfare might remain relevant to health assessment, if it is qualified by a concern for appropriate preference formation. Nevertheless, whilst the malformed preferences objection is not devastating for welfarism, it casts serious doubt upon the moral relevance of the welfarist questions in the SF-36, since the questionnaire contains no means of enquiring into the origins of recipients' preferences. Indeed to do so would reduce the easy administration which its advocates cite in its defence (Ware & Sherbourne 1992, Jenkinson et al. 1993a, 1993b). In effect, then, it presupposes that advantage is in part constituted by actual welfare and is vulnerable to the malformed preferences objection.

Before proceeding to describe a second objection to welfarism, we note a technical problem related to the first objection. It concerns the impact of circumstance not upon desire but judgement, and in particular judgements concerning respondents' general health perception.

The SF-36 seeks information about such judgements when, for example, it asks respondents to report whether their health is "Excellent", "Very good", "Good", "Fair" or "Poor". Such reports, however, may be misleading guides to the relative health of individuals situated in different circumstances. Such will be the case if there exists a positive relationship between enhanced access to medical care, information and literacy, and greater awareness of one's own morbidity. Once again Sen's work is instructive. He notes that

> . . . among the Indian states, Kerala has by a large margin the longest life expectancy at birth (67.5 years for men and 73 years

for women, compared with around 56 years for both men and women in India as a whole), and professional medical assessment gives much evidence of Kerala's successful health transition. And yet Kerala also reports by far the highest rates of self-perceived morbidity (both on the average and in terms of age-specific rates). At the other end are states like Bihar and Uttar Pradesh with very low life expectancy, no evidence of any health transition, and yet astonishingly low rates of self-assessed morbidity. If the medical evidence and the testimony of mortality rates are accepted (and there are no particularly good reasons to rule them out), then the picture of relative morbidity rates as given by self-assessment must be taken to be erroneous (Sen 1993: 134).

Sen's example, if accurate, demonstrates that individuals' judgements, as well as their desires, can be shaped by the circumstances in which they live in a way which jeopardizes their usefulness in making interpersonal comparisons. If, for example, class position plays the same rôle in shaping general health perception within European societies as spatial location allegedly does in India, then the relevance of questions about such perceptions is correspondingly diminished. The value of information about individuals' general health perception is, therefore, dependent upon guarding against such a possibility. The need to do so applies to all subjective modes of assessment in distributive contexts, whether or not they are welfarist. It is, however, to a second objection specifically directed against welfarism that the chapter now turns.

Expensive tastes

The second objection to welfarist standards of interpersonal comparison focuses upon the fact that some people's desires are expensive to satisfy compared with those of others, in the sense that they require a greater share of resources to attain the same level of satisfaction. For illustration of the type of problem this creates, consider the following case popularized by Ronald Dworkin (Dworkin 1981a). Assume that a society seeks to achieve fair shares of welfare, and that this is effected by it ensuring that there exists equality of welfare. Having attained such a state of affairs, suppose now that one individual, Louis, develops a new and expensive ambition, such that he now requires more resources if he is to attain the level of welfare which he previously enjoyed. He might, for example, acquire a passion for fine food and wine, for opera, or for skiing. Suppose also that Louis's new preferences are sincere, and have not been engineered merely to acquire more resources to be spent in attaining a higher degree of satisfaction for his earlier desires. In such circumstances a welfare egalitarian society is committed to providing Louis additional resources to facilitate his pursuit of his new lifestyle, if doing so is necessary to secure equality of welfare. Such a redistribution, however, will strike many as intuitively unfair.

The case of Louis is, therefore, an embarrassment to welfarist standards of comparison. Reflection upon it provides at least *prima facie* grounds to reject subjectivist standards as a means of establishing the relative moral urgency of benefiting distinct individuals. It suggests that the strength of an individual's claim to resources should not vary with changes in her mere preferences. Instead distributive decision-makers should adopt a standard which is more objective, in the sense that it is not as dependent upon the strength of an individual's actual desires. Before explaining the significance of these convictions for the SF-36, it is worth pausing to note the extent to which the previous objection requires the wholesale abandonment of welfarism, or can be assuaged by a modified welfarism.

As with the previous malformed preference objection, an advocate of welfarism might attempt to mollify the expensive tastes objection by modifying her position. In the previous case, that involved gesturing toward an account of healthy preference formation. In response to the case of Louis, one such obvious modification is to suggest that Louis is entitled to additional resources to finance his expensive new ambitions only to the extent that he is not responsible for the acquisition of those preferences. An individual's level of advantage, the welfarist might contend, should not be understood in terms of the amount of welfare actually achieved, but rather the amount to which the individual had access, or the opportunity to enjoy. Pursuing this thought the welfarist might argue as follows. If Louis was responsible for his new ambitions because, for example, he deliberately cultivated them, then his access to welfare remains equal to that of others, even if the amount of welfare which he actually achieved was smaller. Thus, welfare egalitarianism, construed so as to accommodate the importance of personal responsibility, does not endorse the counter-intuitive requirement that Louis's lower level of welfare is a reason to transfer additional resources to him. The adoption of a welfarist standard need not generate unfairness.

A complete assessment of the prospects of modified welfarism is beyond the scope of this chapter. Note, however, that the above suggestion is not without difficulties. For consider another example due to Dworkin, the case of Jude, who initially has modest desires, few resources but an equal level of welfare to others (Dworkin 1981a). He then reads Hemmingway, cultivates a less modest desire to watch bull-fights, and requires an increase in resources to achieve an equal welfare level – but still requires no more resources than others. Dworkin claims many would regard Jude's request for more resources as fair even if he, like Louis, has deliberately acquired an expensive taste. Therefore, we cannot resist Louis's demand on the grounds that he has deliberately cultivated an expensive taste. Modified welfarism is not then an adequate response to the case of Louis. For in supporting resistance to Louis's apparently unreasonable request, it also requires decision-makers to resist the request of Jude, which appears reasonable even though his new preferences have been deliberately acquired.

Reflection upon the previous considerations suggests that problems analogous to those discussed confront at least some aspects of the SF-36, if it is employed as a guide for making distributive decisions. To appreciate their source, note that its rôle limitation components ask individuals not only to assess the extent to which their illness has interfered with their exercise of specific, clearly described actions, such as running or lifting heavy objects. It also asks them to assess its interference with non-specific actions, such as their "work" or their "daily activities". Although such actions are at points described as "normal", it appears that this relates to the extent to which they were *regular actions for the respondent* rather than *typical actions for any individual*. Consequently, it is possible for individuals with the same physical illness, who are capable of performing the same range of bodily movements, to give very different responses about the extent to which their illness has interfered with their normal life and, thus, their level of health status. Such will be the case if the pursuit of their normal lives requires very different physical capabilities.

For illustration, return to the case of Louis, and assume that he now possesses a passion for cross-country skiing, which is expensive not in the demands it makes on his financial endowment (assume Louis lives in an alpine environment and is able to indulge himself regularly and at no great expense): rather skiing is expensive in terms of the demands it makes on an individual's personal endowment of physical abilities. It requires, for example, a degree of physical endurance and agility which greatly exceeds most other regular leisure activities. In contrast Louise's favoured activity, strolling through the park with her dog to visit her brother, is relatively cheap. Thus, if Louis and Louise are both beset by slipped discs they will experience very different degrees of interference even if their physical capacities are roughly equal.

The question then arises about the significance of such a discrepancy to distributive decisions. Does an individual have a stronger claim, other things being equal, to scarce medical treatment to the extent that she suffers from a disease which interferes with the way of life to which she has become accustomed? *Prima facie*, the above criticism of welfarism supports a negative response. The strength of an individual's claim is invariant with the level of subjective dissatisfaction they will undergo if they do not receive additional resources.

Thus, if the above criticism is valid, in estimating the moral urgency of competing claims, physicians should disregard respondents' reports about rôle limitations which they endure because of their illness. They should do so at least where it is probable that respondents have in mind very different rôles when estimating the negative effects of illness. Such could well be the case with the SF-36, given the wide range of activities which might be covered by its rubric concerning "work and other regular activities", "your work or other regular daily activities", and "your normal work (including work both outside the home and housework)". Hence, providing they have the same level of capability, the fact that one patient reports a lower level of satisfaction with her life than another, or a higher degree of illness-induced disruption in her normal life, is not a sound reason to give additional scarce treatment to that individual rather than the other. From the perspective of distributive justice, such facts are not constituents of health status.

To pre-empt misunderstanding, two provisos should now be noted. First, the above conclusion concerned the relative strength of two individuals' claims in a way which disregarded effects upon third parties. Therefore, it would be consistent to accept the conclusion and accept also that, in some cases, interference with regular activities was of relevance to distributive decision-making. Such would be the case if, for example, interference produced benefits for vulnerable third parties, such as dependent children. In such cases, priority might be attached to treating carers over non-carers if doing so was the only means to prevent the occurrence of such harms.

Secondly, and most importantly, the above conclusion is a generalization of an initial objection to welfarist standards of interpersonal comparison. If that expensive tastes objection is invalid, then the objection may be disregarded. As previously noted, considerable debate exists within political philosophy about the force of the objection. This chapter has attempted to explain the significance for subjective health assessment of that debate; it has not attempted to resolve it, although it did note one way in which welfarism might be modified. Its primary purpose will be achieved if readers are convinced that only by addressing such a debate can advocates of subjective health assessment succeed in establishing the relevance to distributive decision-making of its rôle limitation variables.

Note, however, that even if welfarism is defended against the expensive tastes objection in the way suggested, then the value of the SF-36 to distributive decisions remains questionable in two respects. First, the questionnaire is blind to the processes whereby individuals' judgements about their health are formed (or malformed). Secondly, it provides no information about the extent to which they can be held responsible for adopting the activities by reference to which they assess the impact of illness upon their lives. Again a dilemma exists between (a) assuming an unmodified welfarist conception of health status, which is vulnerable to moral objection, or (b) replacing it with a modified account, which makes informational demands that cannot be satisfied by a brief questionnaire.

Capabilities

The previous section assumed that the strength of an individual's claim to resources should not vary with particular subjective states, such as happiness or preference-satisfaction. It concluded that some variables measured by the SF-36 should be disregarded by distributive decision-makers when estimating individuals' relative health status. It suggested, more positively, that such decision-makers should adopt a standard which is more objective. This section pursues that suggestion, and tempers the previous criticism of the SF-36 with more constructive comment.

It examines the questionnaire in the light of Sen's contention that inter-personal comparison should concern individuals' capability to perform, or attain, certain types of function.

Sen's general approach has at least two merits, which are attractive in a standard of interpersonal comparison. First, it is non-fetishistic, since it is concerned with the extent to which individuals are able to make use of particular resources, rather than focusing upon those resources in isola-tion. Secondly, it need not possess the objectionable degree of subjectiv-ity of unmodified welfarist standards (at least so long as the capability to satisfy ones preferences is not included within the set of morally rel-evant functions).

If the appeal to capability is sound, then it appears that the SF-36 is asking at least some appropriate types of question. Such is the case since a number of the variables which it attempts to measure can plausibly be described as capabilities. These include its references to vigorous and moderate physical functions, such as running and moving a table re-spectively, and its references to the incidence of bodily pain. Moreover, such objects are not *mere* capabilities, that is functions of no special moral importance which there is no public duty to protect. The relevance to distributive decisions of these particular capabilities has considerable intuitive plausibility. Unlike, for instance, the capability to ski cross-country, the moral urgency of a claim to public resources based upon the interest in avoiding pain is clearly forceful.

To pre-empt misunderstanding about the compatibility of subjective health assessment and capability approach the following should also be noted. While recognising their importance to distributive decisions, the former in no way depends upon the view that *physical* functionings alone are relevant to assessing an individual's level of advantage. Sen himself has emphasized that importance may be attached to very differ-ent types of capability. These include ones with a psychological and con-ventional dimension such as, for example, "appearing in public without shame" and "taking part in the life of the community" (Sen 1992: 115). Hence, the SF-36's references to the extent to which illness has interfered with "normal social activities with family, friends, neighbours or groups", and "normal work (including work both outside the home and housework)" do not necessarily entail any departure from a capability framework, merely because they eschew an exclusive concern with physical functioning. The previous objection to such questions did not challenge them on this ground. Instead it noted their ambiguity, and suggested this led to a potential unfairness if some individual's particular form of social functioning required substantially more medical resources than others. The solution to this unfairness does not require attending only to physical functions, but rather adopting a more determinate description of normal social functions, which can then form the basis of a claim to medical treatment.

If these observations about the affinity between the capability approach and the SF-36 are correct, then it is appropriate to raise a foundational challenge, which has been directed at Sen's view. It appears equally applicable to subjective health assessment questionnaires which claim moral relevance. The challenge concerns the moral basis for assuming the relevance of some capabilities while denying that of others. What moral reason have distributive decision-makers to ask patients whether their illness has interfered with, for example, their social activities but not with their capability to withstand prolonged immersion in cold water? No attempt will be made here to answer questions such as these (cf. Daniels 1985 and 1990). Note, however, that they cannot be answered merely by observing standard practice, or by reference to the technical properties of subjective health assessment measures. Only by addressing such questions with explicit moral argument can the benefits of those measures be assessed.

Health assessment raises various moral issues, a number of which this chapter has examined. Its main concern has been to highlight neglected ethical problems which arise if welfare information is incorporated within a standard of interpersonal comparison. These problems, however, should not obscure the potential benefits of adopting the patient's point of view in health assessment when questionnaire design is informed by a concern for capability rather than welfare.

Acknowledgement

For instructive comments the authors are grateful to Dr K. Watson and the editor.

CHAPTER 11

Measurement in subjective health assessment: themes and prospects

Crispin Jenkinson, Martin Bardsley and Kate Lawrence

Introduction

This book has addressed issues of measurement that can potentially influence results from health assessment questionnaires. In essence, the message of the text is that methods for the measurement of "health status" currently exist, but that selecting, and, to an even greater extent, designing measures can be a potentially hazardous undertaking. This is due, in part, to methodological problems, such as measurement insensitivity or inappropriate questions being posed, and partly to philosophical problems relating to what it is that should be measured. Terms such as "health status" and "quality of life" tend to be used interchangeably, but, as has been pointed out in this text, could indeed be quite separate phenomena. With no agreement as to definitions, and with no "gold standard", subjective health measurement could stand accused of lacking direction. This book has attempted to highlight some of the issues surrounding both theoretical issues and methodological problems.

The increasingly widespread belief that traditional morbidity and mortality measures are insufficient to capture the full impact of medical interventions, and the accelerating rate at which new treatments and pharmaceutical products are being developed, have brought with them increasing interest in the measurement of quality of life or health status. In 1977 Quality of Life became a "keyword" by which articles could be retrieved by the U.S. National Library of Medicine MEDLINE Computer Search System. The number of questionnaires that have been developed has increased dramatically, and the number of scientific papers reporting results from studies that have attempted in some way to measure what is variously called "quality of life", "health status", "health related quality of life", and "subjective health state" has grown exponentially. In order to place some form on this large and increasingly disparate field, a number of texts have attempted to document validated existing measures (McDowell & Newell 1987, Bowling 1991, Wilkin et al. 1992, 1993), to provide outlines of uses of such measures (Teeling-Smith 1988, Stewart & Walker 1988). This text is complementary to such volumes as it has attempted to address a number of the methodological considerations of which potential users of questionnaires should be aware. It is now increasingly agreed that data concerning quality of life can provide potentially invaluable information concerning the impact of medical interventions.

Benefits of health assessment

The "potentially invaluable" information that can be made available from health measures falls into a number of different categories. At one level health measurement profiles can be used in clinical research as outcome measures in randomized controlled trials. Data can be gained from patients regarding their health status, and this can be used to determine whether one treatment has proved more successful than another or a placebo treatment in terms of self-reported quality of life. At another level health status measures can be used to evaluate ongoing clinical practice. This may be on individual patients, or groups. For example it has been suggested that health status data can act as an adjunct to the standard clinical interview, and may be useful for informing medical practitioners of the wellbeing of individual patients in their care. It has been argued that this is one of the most worthwhile features of the Dartmouth COOP Charts, a health measurement questionnaire designed for use in family practice (Nelson et al. 1990). Studies suggest that both patients and clinicians believe the use of the charts has led to improved interaction, and better treatment (Beaufait et al. 1992). On a group analysis level, Ellwood (1988) has advocated the use of health measurement questionnaires routinely in clinical practice to evaluate the impact of medical care upon specific groups. The Health Outcomes Institute in America is encouraging providers to administer questionnaires to groups of patients who will be followed through treatment and beyond.

There is some interest in using these questionnaires as part of clinical audit programmes in the UK, to assist clinicians in monitoring the outcomes of care. It is also possible to monitor not the treatment regime *per se*, but the providers of the treatment. Subjective health assessment measures have been advocated as a method of evaluating the effect of different methods of providing health care and to assess the impact of cost-containment strategies. This was the main thrust of the work undertaken in the Medical Outcomes Study in America, which was the first major project to use patient-assessed data to evaluate variations in health care provision (Tarlov et al. 1989). Of course it is possible to monitor not only groups of patients over time, but whole districts. Population mortality statistics provide only limited information about the health of general populations in the developed countries and the use of standardized health assessment measures may have a use in monitoring the health of whole towns, regions or countries or of social groups within them (Ware 1992).

Essentially, data from health status measurement can be used to improve knowledge of treatments, to provide an indication of ill health in specific groups in population surveys, and as a basis for determining efficient allocation of resources for health care. However, this text has highlighted the problems that exist in undertaking these tasks. Not all questionnaires are appropriate in all settings, for all purposes or for all respondents. Researchers and clinicians set upon including quality of life measurement in practice or in research studies must consider carefully exactly what they are trying to determine by using health status measures. As Ray Fitzpatrick has pointed out in this volume, the Nottingham Health Profile would be an inappropriate measure to determine need in a population sample, as most respondents score zero on this questionnaire, and hence ill health is under-reported. Similarly, other questionnaires, such as the Functional Limitations Profile, would be inappropriate for ongoing routine evaluation of medical care due to the length of the instrument. As Kathy Rowan has pointed out, questionnaires such as the Dartmouth COOP Charts, the SF-6, and, indeed single item measures, are more appropriate for routine settings. What is lost in precision and reliability when questionnaires become so brief is perhaps less than one might expect. Furthermore, patients are capable of assessing changes in health status over time both directly and in a way that, at least when compared with other clinical data, seems accurate. As yet there is only a limited amount of research available on the extent to which patients can evaluate changes in health directly. Instead research in the area has been primarily concerned with the assessment of change between two separate subjective evaluations. However, Sue Ziebland provides a convincing case that questions directly requesting patients to evaluate changes in their health can provide meaningful information quickly and economically. While many complex forms of weighting and deriving questionnaires have been suggested, there is still much to be said for more simple measures, providing that the questions are asked in a standardized manner. Furthermore, the sensitivity and complexity required in an instrument depends on the clinical context in which it is being used. Major impairment will be detected even by a relatively insensitive measure. For example, if a patient is unable to walk after a hip replacement this may be detected by a fairly crude measure. However more subtle changes, such as those achieved by some drug treatments for arthritis, may require a more sensitive instrument.

Further work is required to establish what change in the available measures can be regarded as clinically important. The change score obtained will depend on the responsiveness of the instrument as much as it depends on the change in health being assessed. In some circumstances a measure could be regarded as too sensitive, if it is measuring a change that is not clinically, or indeed subjectively, relevant. An oversensitive measure may produce large change scores even when used to assess interventions that produce effects so small as to be clinically, or subjectively, unimportant. Undeniably, the production of such measures would obviously be a good way of marketing drug treatments!

One of the most important steps in choosing a scale is identifying health changes that are to be expected as a result of any given health care intervention. While it may be generally agreed that improving quality of life is in itself a worthy endeavour, the way this will be manifested will vary considerably according to the patient group and the service offered. One way to overcome which domains are appropriate to given patient groups, and, indeed, individuals, may be overcome by asking patients directly what aspects of their life have been affected and to what extent. Is such a procedure possible and appropriate? The chapters by Ruta and Garratt, and Clayton and Williams address some of the most complex issues in this area. In essence they starkly contrast two strongly held views within this field, for there are those who believe "quality of life" can be both defined and measured, and those who see the term as vague and virtually useless, and, furthermore, not the domain to which the medical profession should address itself. Danny Ruta and his colleagues have attempted to tackle difficult philosophical issues in an empirical manner, while Matthew Clayton and Andrew Williams have attempted to delimit the extent to which an enquiry into the "quality of life", could go. It is not, argue Clayton and Williams, for the medical profession to improve "quality of life", in terms of "happiness" or "overall wellbeing", *per se*, but rather to improve the capabilities of individuals such that they are in a position to live a life with quality. Ruta and Garratt, in contrast, see the quality of an individual's life as potentially adversely affected by ill health. The confounding of expectations from reality, as caused by health-related problems, is that which acts so as to reduce the quality of one's existence. Although they would be the first to argue that the medical profession is no universal panacea providing for all the needs of all individuals, they do see medical treatment as potentially improving health-related quality of life. Thus, they argue, medical care should be evaluated not in terms of whether it increases the capabilities of individuals but whether it actually directly improves quality of life. However, what makes for quality of life is distinct to each individual, and as such measurement should address itself as much as possible to gaining highly individualized data from respondents. Patients, individually, thus nominate areas of their lives which have been adversely affected by their health state, and indicate the extent of this impact. The results from each of the items selected is then aggregated to produce a single index figure. Such a procedure has the advantage of not imposing pre-existing definitions of health state upon respondents (Ruta et al. in press, a). Research in this area has been undertaken with patients undergoing hip replacement (McGee et al. 1992, O'Boyle et al. 1992), back pain (Ruta, in press, a) and arthritis (Tugwell et al. 1987, 1990). Such methods are, like many of the other means of deriving single index figures, still in their infancy and hence not widely applied. A number of issues need to be addressed, such as whether respondents should select new dimensions each time they complete the questionnaire in longitudinal studies, whether aggregating unrelated dimensions is appropriate, and whether patients should select dimensions from a list (which perhaps contradicts the whole philosophy of this approach), or simply select from any areas they think important. Such issues are at present receiving attention from a number of researchers, and while the generalized application of this new technique seems a long way off, it is undeniably an interesting and potentially worthwhile new approach to the whole field of subjective health measurement, and throws up as many questions as it does answers.

Methodological considerations

As this text has highlighted, choosing a health status measure, or designing one, is not as straightforward a task as might initially seem to be the
case. A number of issues must be considered when designing a questionnaire. Instruments must be reliable, valid and sensitive to change. Questionnaires must be reliable over time. Thus, they should produce the
same, or very similar results, on two or more administrations to the
same respondents, provided, of course, there is good reason to believe
that the health status of the patients has not changed. The difficulty with
such a method of validating a questionnaire is that it is often uncertain
as to whether results that may indicate a questionnaire is unreliable are
in fact no more than a product of real change in health status. Due to the
potential difficulties in gaining an accurate picture of reliability in this
way, many researchers adopt the Cronbach's alpha statistic (Cronbach
1951), to determine internal reliability. Internal reliability refers to the
extent to which items on a scale are tapping a single underlying construct, and therefore there is a high level of inter-item correlation.
Assuming that such high levels of inter-item correlation are not a product of chance it is commonplace to assume that a high alpha statistic
indicates the questionnaire is tapping an underlying construct and
hence is reliable. There is, however, disagreement as to whether such a
method can be viewed as appropriate for assuming a questionnaire is reliable over time (Sheldon 1993, Ruta et al. 1993).

When selecting measures, researchers and clinicians must select measures that are valid, i.e. reliably measuring that which they are intended
to measure. While many questionnaires are advocated as "reliable" or
"psychometrically sound" it would be naïve to assume that such measures are either perfect in themselves, or perfect for all uses. For a measure to be "reliable" and produce "valid" results it must be used with
appropriate consideration to its own qualities and attributes. Textbooks
tend to write aspects of validity as if they were properties inherent in
questionnaires, and hence never influenced by conditions external to
them. This is simply not the case. For example, face validity refers to
whether items on a questionnaire superficially appear to make sense,
and can be easily understood. This may seem a simple enough test for a
questionnaire to pass, but, for example, place of completion can potentially influence the meaning of questionnaires. Thus while a questionnaire may appear to make sense when the researcher reads it in a library,

it may make considerably less sense when a patient is completing it in hospital. As Sue Ziebland has noted in her chapter some items on the FLP can be influenced by place of administration. It has been suggested that individuals are more likely to affirm certain statements when in hospital than elsewhere. For example, items such as "I stay in bed most of the day" are more likely to be affirmed in hospital than, for example, at home, though the need to stay in bed in hospital may be induced by hospital requirements rather than by state of health *per se* (Ziebland et al. 1992, Jenkinson et al. 1993d). Thus, when choosing a measure it is vital to check items to determine whether it will make appropriate sense to those who are likely to be completing it. Indeed, piloting the chosen questionnaire, and asking respondents how they have interpreted the questions may be an appropriate strategy. Simon Williams, in his chapter on the FLP, highlights some of the methodological problems that can be encountered with this instrument, which, despite its imperfections, tends to be viewed as something of a "gold standard".

It is important to note that subjective health measurement questionnaires are not designed to be used as substitutes for traditional measures of clinical endpoints. On the contrary, they are intended to complement existing measures and to provide a fuller picture of health state than can be gained by medical measures alone. However, to be useful such measures must be carefully chosen. The wrong choice of measure could produce meaningless or misleading data. Due to errors of design, analysis or administration, questionnaires may produce data that make ill people seem healthy and vice versa.

Single index figures of health status appeal to those who wish to compare different treatments and interventions. However, while such single index figures give the impression of comparability between illness states and treatments they may do so unfairly. For example, one standardized health index measure, the Euroqol (Euroqol Group 1990) questionnaire does not contain a dimension evaluating sleep disturbance, and a treatment aimed primarily at improving this dimension of health may not appear to have been efficacious if assessed by this measure.

Single index figures gained from patient-generated measures, such as those outlined by Ruta and Garratt in this volume and O'Boyle et al. (1992) may overcome the above criticism. Essentially the dimensions chosen by patients are seen as paramount, and so if a patient is primarily concerned about the impact of illness on their sleep patterns, this will be incorporated in the measure. However, difficulties arise here. At initial interview a patient may claim their quality of life in five areas is affected. At follow up, these areas may have improved, so if the patient completes the questionnaire using the same dimensions chosen at time one an improvement in health status will be apparent. However, side effects of drug treatment may have influenced other aspects of the respondent's life, and the patient's overall quality of life may not have improved at all. When using such a measure it is therefore appropriate to also include a generic instrument so as to ensure as wide as possible coverage of health-related dimensions.

Generic measures, such as the FLP, the SF-36 Health Survey Questionnaire and the NHP, indicate clearly which dimensions of health status are being measured, but the dimensions included may not be appropriate in the assessment of every intervention. For example, the FLP, despite having 12 dimensions, lacks a specific category measuring pain. Results from generic measures can, of course, be compared with data from other populations and illness groups. For example, normative data can be used to compare the health status of a particular patient group with that of the general population (Ware 1993). However, it is still important that disease specific measures, such as the Health Assessment Questionnaire (Fries et al. 1982) – developed to measure health status in patients with rheumatoid arthritis – are used alongside such generic measures, since disease specific measures are, by their very nature, likely to tap particular aspects of ill health that are unique to particular illnesses.

Ceiling and floor effects must be considered. The NHP has been criticized because it detects only the severe end of ill health, and thus most respondents score zero on many, if not all, of the six dimensions of the questionnaire (Kind & Carr-Hill 1987). The items on the questionnaire were chosen to represent severe health states, and so individuals who have mild to moderate illness may not be detected with this instrument. In a study of change over time, respondents with minor ailments may improve, but if their initial score on dimensions of the NHP was zero, such improvement may not be detected (floor effect). As Lucie Wright notes in her chapter the SF-36 was a response to problems found in a previous instrument developed from the RAND studies, the SF-20. However, due to insensitivity to those with serious illnesses, the questionnaire had to be refined and developed. Respondents on the SF-20 could score as maximally ill on the questionnaire, yet the extent of their illness state was not fully reflected in the questionnaire. Such severely ill respondents fall beyond the measurement range. Thus, while these patients may improve over time, it is still possible they may continue to score as maximally ill on the questionnaire (ceiling effect). Such floor and ceiling effects are more likely to be found on instruments with small numbers of items (Bindman et al. 1990). Similarly, questionnaires which contain compressed response ranges may not be sensitive to change. Take, for example, an item such as "How do you feel today?". This question could indicate very different amounts of change depending on whether the response categories were "Excellent, Very Good, Good, Fair, Poor" or "Good, Fair, Poor, Very Poor, Terrible". Someone who viewed their health state as having improved from terrible to poor is unlikely to show change on the first response set. Similarly, someone who viewed their health state as having been excellent at the first interview, but good at the second, may not show change if administered the second response format.

Related to floor and ceiling effects is another important aspect of health status measures: sensitivity to change or "responsiveness". For health status measures to be useful in evaluating the impact of medical interventions they must be "sensitive". It is thus imperative, when selecting a measure, to determine the exact nature of the questions asked and the time scales utilized. For example, a questionnaire such as the NHP, designed to tap the extreme end of ill health, is unlikely to be sensitive to small changes in health status among patients with minor illnesses.

Furthermore, in longitudinal studies it is important that the mode of administration of questionnaires is kept consistent. For example, due to the nature of some of the items in the FLP, respondents may gain higher scores in hospital than as outpatients or when at home, and such scores may not actually reflect health state. Items such as "I stay in bed more" are more likely to be affirmed in hospital, and may not accurately reflect the impact of the illness *per se* on a person's life

Conclusion

Health status measures can provide a useful adjunct to the data traditionally obtained from mortality and morbidity statistics, or from traditional clinical and laboratory assessments. However, careful consideration must be given to the choice of measures. At best, however, health status measures may permit scientific questions to be answered fully in the context of clinical trials, and, in time, they may find their way into routine use. However, the results obtained from such measures must be made intuitive and meaningful to clinicians, as well as to researchers, and adequate care must be taken to ensure appropriate measures tapping relevant domains are being utilized. Subjective health status measurement could provide much needed data on the impact of clinical interventions on the day-to-day lives of patients; done without due care of the pitfalls, however, such data could be irrelevant, or even worse, misleading.

Glossary

alpha   A statistic used to determine the internal reliability of scales (see reliability).

ceiling and floor effects   Refer to the response range and the method of scoring an instrument. Thus an instrument, applied to a random sample of the population, which is not sensitive to lower levels of ill health and that is scored from 0 (good health) to 100 (poor health) would be said to manifest a floor effect, as most respondents would score zero. On the other hand if the instrument was scored from 0 (poor health) to 100 (good health) this would be referred to as a ceiling effect, as most respondents would score 100. Such floor and ceiling effects are more likely to be found in instruments with small numbers of items.

clinical trial   An experiment to assess the efficacy of a treatment.

cost–utility analysis   A form of economic cost–effectiveness analysis where the effects of health care interventions are assessed according to the quality adjusted life years gained or lost (see QALY).

dimensions of health   Theoretically or empirically distinct aspects of health, for example physical and mental health.

domain   See dimensions of health.

effect size   A statistic for determining the difference between scores gained at two different times. This statistic has been recommended by Kazis et al. (1989) as a method of evaluating the sensitivity of health measurement instruments to important clinical change, calculated by dividing the mean change in score by the baseline standard deviation.

floor effect   See ceiling and floor effects.

generic measure   A measure which is designed for use with any illness groups or population samples, as opposed to those intended for specific illness groups.

health   There are numerous definitions of health, but perhaps the most widely quoted is that of the World Health Organisation, "a state of complete physical, mental, and social wellbeing and not merely the absence of disease or infirmity" (WHO 1948).

health index   Where all the items of an instrument are summed producing one overall score, for example the Euroquol (Euroquol Group 1990).

health outcomes   The end results of medical interventions and processes. These can be assessed in terms of mortality, morbidity, physiological measures and, increasingly, more subjective patient-based assessments of health.

health profile   A questionnaire covering various dimensions of health, as opposed to a health index which sums all measured aspects of health into a single figure.

health-related quality of life   This refers to an individual's level of health-related wellbeing. Measurement of health-related quality of life addresses the various dimensions of health (see dimensions of health).

health status   A level of health in terms of physical, social and mental wellbeing.

instrument   The tool with which health status or quality of life is measured, usually in the form of a questionnaire.

internal consistency   See reliability.

item   An individual question which may stand alone or form part of a battery of questions in a dimension.

item content   Refers to the actual wording of the individual questions. Such content must at least satisfy requirements of face validity (see validity).

longitudinal study   Where individuals in a study are followed over time.

multidimensional measures   Instruments which consider health in more than one dimension/domain, of health; for example mobility, pain, mental health.

non-parametric methods   Statistical analyses which assume that data does not follow the "normal distribution".

normative data   Data which are representative of a population.

parametric methods   Statistical analyses in which the data are assumed to be normally distributed.

precision   The ability of an instrument to differentiate between illness groups, or states of health.

QALY (quality-adjusted life year)   A generic measure of health benefit which attempts to represent the relative value attached by society to different improvements in health enabling systematic comparison between a variety of health care interventions. Comparisons between treatment programmes are expressed in quality-adjusted life years (see Williams & Kind 1992). With both a measure of the life years gained from a particular intervention and of the quality of life in each of those years it is possible to calculate the number of QALYs obtained. Thus an index of quality of life, multiplied by the number of years in that health state equals the number of QALYs.

random sample   Where each individual in the given population has an equal chance of selection into the sample.

reliability   A reliable measure is one which produces consistent results from the same subjects at different times when there exists no evidence of change.

test-retest reliability   This involves the administration of an instrument on two separate occasions to the same population. The correlation between scores provides an estimate of the measure's reliability. The two occasions need to be far enough apart so that previous responses cannot be remembered but close enough in time so that change in the true score is minimal.

internal consistency   Assessment of internal consistency involves examining the extent to which a number of items addressing the same concept actually are doing so. There are a number of ways of calculating the correlation between items, for example: split-half reliability – whereby the measure is randomly split into two groups and reliability is assessed by the correlation between the two half tests, and Cronbach's Alpha – a statistical test of internal consistency based on the mean correlation between items.

inter-rater reliability   Addresses the consistency of a measure when administered by different interviewers. This is tested by interviewing the same people with the same measures but using different interviewers with only a short period of time between. Kappa coefficient of agreement is the statistical tool used to assess whether differences were due to agreement or chance.

response range   The set of answers available to respondents for each item.

responsiveness   The extent to which an instrument can detect change in health status over time. (See also ceiling and floor effects).

scales   A graded system of categories, of which there are broadly 4 types outlined below:

nominal scales   These scales distinguish classes of objects. For example, the classification of sex into 1 = male and 2 = female is a nominal scale. A more complex nominal scale is the International Classification of Diseases, where numerical values classify all diagnoses and presenting problems. There is no hierarchy implied by the values ascribed, so in the example of sex it would be equally as valid to code 1 = female and 2 = male. Statistical analysis of such data must be restricted to simple cross tabulations and frequencies.

ordinal scales   Classes or objects are ordered on a continuum (for example, from Best to Worst). No indication is given as to the distance between values, although a hierarchy is assumed to exist. Thus when classifying an illness into 1 = mild, 2 = moderate and 3 = severe it cannot be assumed that the extent of difference between mild and moderate is similar to the difference between moderate and severe. Rank order correlation is an appropriate statistical analysis for such data. Tabular representation of data is appropriate but even simple descriptive statistics (such as means, and standard deviations) based on such data should be avoided as results can be misleading.

interval scales   It is assumed that data on an interval scale is ordered, and the distances between values on one part of the scale are equal in distance to the distances between values on another part of the scale. Temperature is measured on such a scale. However, interval scales lack an absolute baseline anchor point. For example, a thermometer is an interval scale but it is not possible to assume that 60°F is twice as hot as 30°F. Subtraction and addition of such data are appropriate, but not division or multiplication. Pearson correlation, factor analysis and discriminant analysis are appropriate analysis techniques.

ratio scales   A ratio scale is an interval scale with an absolute zero point, so that ratios between values can be meaningfully defined. Thus time, weight and height are all examples of ratio scales. For example, it is perfectly acceptable to assume that 30 seconds is twice as long a time period as 60 seconds. All forms of statistical analysis may be used with such data, although care should be taken in choice of methods depending on the spread of the data (see parametric methods and non-parametric methods).

sensitivity An instrument's ability to detect change over time.

standardized response mean A statistic for determining the difference between scores gained at two different times. It is calculated by dividing the mean change on a scale by the mean change in the standard deviation. Such a method is recommended when comparing the sensitivity to change of various health status measures (Katz et al. 1992). See also effect size.

subjective wellbeing The patient's assessment of their own health status as opposed to professionally or clinically defined indicators.

Thurstone's method of paired comparisons A technique for gaining relative values for items on a questionnaire. Thus on the NHP the item "I cannot walk at all" gains greater value than "I have difficulty walking about outside". See McKenna et al. (1981) for a full discussion of the procedure for calculating weights for the NHP, or Steiner & Norman (1989) for an outline of the general procedures of Thurstone scaling.

validity The extent to which an indicator measures the desired underlying concept. There are various steps in the validation process from which to establish how confident one is that the scale or item is measuring the desired attribute:

face validity The need for a questionnaire to apparently tap, simply by item content, an underlying dimension. Questions should be unambiguous and easily understood, and should reflect issues appropriate to the dimension.

content validity The extent to which items on a questionnaire tap all the relevant aspects of the attribute they are intending to measure.

criterion validity The extent to which a measure correlates with a pre-existing one, preferably a "gold standard". There are two types:

　　concurrent validity Where a new measure is administered at the same time as a pre-existing one, and the two are correlated.

　　predictive validity The predictive power of a given instrument against some other measure. For example, instruments to predict the weather can be validated by how correct they are in their predictions.

construct validity Where hypotheses are generated and a questionnaire tested to determine if it actually reflects these prior hypotheses. For example, the construct validity of the SF-36 has been checked to ensure that certain groups (e.g. older, lower social classes, those with illnesses) gain lower scores than other groups (e.g. younger, higher social classes, those without illnesses).

convergent and discriminant validity A measure should both converge with other indicators of the same concept and be able to discriminate unrelated indicators.

weighting Items which are given values indicating their relative importance to other items on a scale are said to be weighted. For example, on the NHP, the item "I cannot walk at all" is given a greater value than "I need help to walk about outside".

References

Aaronson, N. K., C. Acquadro, J. Alonso, et al. 1992. International quality of life assessment (IQOLA) project. *Quality of Life Research* 1, 349–51.

Aday, L. 1989. *Designing and conducting health surveys*. San Francisco: Jossey-Bass.

Age Concern 1974. *The attitudes of the retired and the elderly*. London: National old people's welfare council.

Ahmad, W. I., E. E. Kernohan, M. R. Baker 1989. Influence of ethnicity and unemployment on the perceived health of a sample of general practice attenders. *Community Medicine* 11, 148–56.

Albert, D., R. Munson, M. D. Resnik 1988. *Reasoning in medicine: An introduction to clinical inference*. Baltimore: The Johns Hopkins University Press.

Albrecht, G. 1992. *The disability business: Rehabilitation in America*. London: Sage.

Albrecht, G. L. 1976. Socialization and the disability process. In *The sociology of physical disability and rehabilitation*, G. L. Albrecht (ed.), 3–38. Pittsburgh: University of Pittsburgh Press.

Albrecht, G. L. 1973. Agents of social change and social conflict in developing countries; indigenous health professionals and paraprofessionals in Iran and Kenya. Paper presented at the Southern Sociological Association, New Orleans.

Albrecht, G. L. & P. C. Higgins 1977. Rehabilitation success: the interrelationships of multiple criteria. *Journal of Health and Social Behavior* 18, 36–45.

Albrecht, G. L. & J. A. Levy 1991. Chronic illness and disability as life course events. In *Advances in medical sociology volume II: Chronic disease across the lifecourse*, G. L. Albrecht & J. A. Levy (eds), 3–16. Greenwich, Connecticut: JAI press.

Altman, D. 1991. *Practical statistics for medical research*. London: Chapman & Hall.

Andrews, F. M. & S. B. Withy 1976. *Social indicators of well-being: America's perception of life quality*. New York: Plenum.

Anspach, R. R. 1991. Everyday methods for assessing organizational effectiveness. *Social Forces* 38, 1–19.

Antonovsky, A. 1993. The structure and properties of the sense of coherence scale. *Social Science and Medicine* 36, 725–33.

191

Applegate, W., J. Blass, T. Williams 1990. Instruments for the functional assessment of older patients. *New England Journal of Medicine* **322**, 1207–14.

Arneson, R. 1990. Liberalism, distributive subjectivism, and equality of opportunity for welfare. *Philosophy and Public Affairs* **19**, 158–94.

Arrow, K. 1973. Some ordinalist-utilitarian notes on Rawls' theory of justice. *Journal of Philosophy* **70**, 245–63.

Bardsley, M. J., C. W. Venables, J. Watson, J. Goodfellow, P. D. Wright 1992. Evidence for the validity of a health status measure in assessing short term outcomes in cholecystectomy. *Quality in Health Care* **1**, 10–14.

Bassett, S. S., J. Magaziner, J. R. Hebel 1990. Reliability of proxy response on mental health indices for aged, community-dwelling women. *Psychology of Aging* **2**, 127–32.

Baum, M., T. Priestman, R. R. West, E. M. Jones 1980. A comparison of subjective responses in a trial comparing endocrine with cytotoxic treatment in advanced carcinoma of the breast. *European Journal of Cancer* **16**, Supplement 1, 223–6.

Beaufait, D. W., E. C. Nelson, J. M. Landgraf, et al. 1992. COOP measures of functional status. In *Tools for primary care research, research methods for primary care, Volume 2*, M. Stewart, F. Tudiver, M. J. Bass, E. V. Dunn, P. G. Norton (eds), 151–68. London: Sage.

Beck, A., C. Ward, M. Mendelson, J. Mock, J. Erbaugh 1961. An inventory for measuring depression. *Archives of General Psychiatry* **4**, 561–71.

Becker, M., M. D. Diamond, F. Sainfort 1993. A new client centered index for measuring quality of life in persons with severe and persistent mental illness. Unpublished paper, Madison, Wisconsin.

Bergner, M. 1988. Development, testing, and use of the Sickness Impact Profile. In *Quality of life: assessement and application*, S. R. Walker & R. M. Rosser (eds), 79–93. Lancaster: MTP Press.

Bergner, M. 1985. Measurement of health status. *Medical Care* **23**, 696–704.

Bergner, M., R. A. Bobbitt, S. Kressel, et al. 1976a. The Sickness Impact Profile: conceptual formulation and methodology for the development of a health status measure. *International Journal of Health Services* **6**, 393–415.

Bergner, M., R. A. Bobbitt, W. E. Pollard, D. P. Martin, B. S. Gilson 1976b. The Sickness Impact Profile: validation of a health status measure. *Medical Care* **14**, 57–67.

Bergner, M., R. A. Bobbitt, with W. B. Carter, B. S. Gilson 1981. The Sickness Impact Profile: development and final version of a health status measure. *Medical Care* **19**, 787–805.

Bergner, L., A. P. Hallstrom, M. Bergner, et al. 1985. Health status of survivors of cardiac arrest and of myocardial infarction controls. *American Journal of Public Health* **75**, 1321–3.

Bergner, M., L. D. Hudson, D. A. Conrad, et al. 1988. The cost and efficacy of home care for patients with chronic lung disease. *Medical Care* **26**, 566–79.

Bergner M. & M. L. Rothman 1987. Health status measures: an overview and guide for selection. *Annual Review of Public Health* **8**, 191–210.

Bindman A. B., D. Keane, N. Lurie 1990. Measuring health changes among severely ill patients: the floor phenomenon. *Medical Care* **28**, 1142–52.

Birren, J. E. 1993. Measuring quality of life in old age. Paper presented at the XV International Congress of Gerontology, Budapest, Hungary.

Black, N., M. Pettigrew, K. McPherson 1993. Comparison of NHS and private patients undergoing elective transurethral resection of the prostate for benign prostatic hypertrophy. *Quality in Health Care* **2**, 11–16.

Blaxter, M. 1990. *Health and lifestyles*. London: Tavistock-Routledge.

Blaxter, M. 1985. Self definition of health status and consulting rates in primary care. *Quarterly Journal of Social Affairs* **1**, 131–71.

Blazer, D. & J. Houpt 1979. Perception of poor health in the healthy older adult. *Journal of the American Geriatrics Society* **27**, 330–34.

Bowling, A. 1991. *Measuring health: a review of quality of life measurement scales*. Milton Keynes: Open University Press.

Brazier, J. E., R. Harper, N. M. B. Jones, et al. 1992. Validating the SF-36 health survey questionnaire: new outcome measure for primary care. *British Medical Journal* **305**, 160–64.

Brewer, J. & A. Hunter 1989. *Multimethod research*. Newbury Park: Sage Publications.

Brook R. H., J. E. Ware, W. H. Rogers et al. 1983. Does free care improve adults' health? Results from a randomized control trial. *New England Journal of Medicine* **309**, 1426–34.

Brown, J. H., M. D. Lewis, E. Kazis, et al. 1984. The dimensions of health outcomes: a cross validated examination of health status measurement. *American Journal of Public Health* **74**, 159–61.

Bruusgaard, D., I. Nessioy, O. Rutle, K. Furuseth, B. Natvig. Measuring functional status in a population survey. The Dartmouth COOP functional health assessment charts/WONCA used in an epidemiological study. *Family Practice* **10**, 212–18.

Bury, M. 1991. The sociology of chronic illness: a review of research and prospects. *Sociology of Health and Illness* **13**, 451–68.

Bury, M. 1982. Chronic illness as biographical disruption. *Sociology of Health and Illness* **4**, 167–82.

Buxton M. 1983. The economics of heart transplant programmes: measuring the benefits. In *Measuring the social benefits of medicine*, G. Teeling-Smith (ed.). London: Office of Health Economics.

Byrne, M. 1992. Cancer chemotherapy and quality of life. *British Medical Journal* **304**, 1523–4.

Calkins, D. R., L. V. Rubenstein, P. D. Cleary, et al. 1991. Failure of physicians to recognise functional disability in ambulatory patients. *Annals of Internal Medicine* **114**, 451–4.

Calman, K. C. 1984. Quality of life in cancer patients – an hypothesis. *Journal of Medical Ethics* **10**, 124–7.

Campbell, A., P. Converse, W. Rodgers 1976. *The quality of American life*. New York: Russell Sage.

Carr-Hill, R. 1989. Assumptions of the QALY procedure. *Social Science & Medicine* **29**, 469–81.

Chambers, L. W., M. Haight, G. Norman, et al. 1987. Sensitivity to change and the effect of mode of administration on health status measurement. *Medical Care* **25**, 470–79.

Chambers, L. W., L. A. MacDonald, P. Tugwell, et al. 1982. The McMaster health index questionnaire as a measure of quality of life for patients with rheumatoid disease. *Journal of Rheumatology* **9**, 780–84.

Chambers, L. W., D. L. Sackett, C. Goldsmith, et al. 1976. Development and application of an index of social function. *Health Service Research* **11**, 430–41.

Charlton, J. R. H., D. L. Patrick, H. Peach 1983. Use of multi-variate measures of disability in health surveys. *Journal of Epidemiology and Community Health* **37**, 296–304.

Cleary, P. 1991. *Patient functioning and satisfaction questionnaire for patients with chest pain.* Boston: Harvard University.

Cleary, P. D., S. Edgmen-Levitan, M. Roberts, et al. 1991. Patients evaluate their hospital care; a national survey. *Health Affairs* **10**, 254–67.

Cohen, C. 1982. On the quality of life: some philosophical reflections. *Circulation* **66**, Supplement 3, 29–33.

Cohen, G. A. 1989. On the currency of egalitarian justice. *Ethics* **99**, 906–44.

Cohen, J. 1977. *Statistical power for the behavioural sciences.* New York: Academic Press.

Cook, T. D. & D. T. Campbell 1979. *Quasi-experimentation: design and analysis issues for field settings.* Chicago: Rand McNally.

Cox, D., R. Fitzpatrick, A. Fletcher et al. 1992. Quality of life assessment: can we keep it simple? *Journal of the Royal Statistical Society.* Series A **155**, 353–93.

Cronbach, L. J. 1951. Coefficient alpha and the internal structure of tests. *Psychometrica* **16**, 297–334.

Croog, S., S. Levine, M. Testa, et al. 1986. The effects of antihypertensive therapy on the quality of life. *New England Journal of Medicine* **314**, 1657–64.

Curtis, S. 1987. Self reported morbidity in London and Manchester: inter-urban and intra-urban variations. *Social Indicators Research* **19**, 255–72.

Dalkey, N. C., D. L. Rourke, R. Lewis, et al. 1972. *Studies in the quality of life – delphi and decision-making.* Massachusetts: Lexington.

Daniels, N. 1990. Equality of what?: Welfare, resources, or capabilities? *Philosophy and Phenomenological Research* **50**, Supplement, 273–96.

Daniels, N. 1985. *Just Health Care.* Cambridge: Cambridge University Press.

Daut R. L., C. S. Cleeland, R. C. Flannery 1983. Development of the Wisconsin Brief Pain Questionnaire to assess pain in cancer and other diseases. *Pain* **17**, 197–210.

de Bruin, A. F., L. P. de Witte, F. Stevens, J. P. M. Diederiks 1993. Sickness Impact Profile: the state of the art of a generic functional status measure. *Social Science and Medicine* **35**, 1003–14.

Dean, K. J. 1993. Self-care and health promotion. Paper presented at the International Congress of Gerontology, Budapest, Hungary.

DeLame, P. A., A. M. Droussin, M. Thomso, L. Verhaest, S. Wallace 1989. The effects of Enalapril on hypertension and quality of life. A large multicentre study in Belgium. *Acta Cardiologica* **44**, 289–302.

Department of Health 1992. *Assessing the effects of health technologies.* London:

Department of Health.

Devins, G., S. Edworthy, P. Seland, et al. 1993. Differences in illness intrusiveness across rheumatoid arthritis, end-stage renal disease, and multiple sclerosis. *Journal of Nervous and Mental Disease* **181**, 377–81.

Deyo, R. A. 1988. Measuring the quality of life of patients with rheumatoid arthritis. In *Quality of life: assessment and application*, S. R. Walker & R. M. Rosser (eds), 205–21. Lancaster: MTP Press.

Deyo, R. A. 1986. Comparative validity of the Sickness Impact Profile and shorter scales for functional assesment in low back pain. *Spine* **11**, 951–4.

Deyo, R. A. & A. K. Diehl 1983. Measuring physical and psychosocial function in patients with low back pain. *Spine* **8**, 635–42.

Deyo, R. A. & T. Inui 1984. Towards clinical applications of health status measures: sensitivity of scales to clinically important changes. *Health Services Research* **19**, 275–89.

Deyo, R. A., T. S. Inui, J. D. Leininger, S. Overman 1982. Physical and psychosocial function in rheumatoid arthritis: clinical use of a self-administered health status instrument. *Archives of Internal Medicine* **142**, 879–82.

Deyo, R. A., T. S. Inui, J. D. Leininger, S. S. Overman 1983. Measuring functional outcomes in chronic disease: a comparison of traditional scales and a self-administered health status questionnaire in patients with rheumatoid arthritis. *Medical Care* **21** (2), 180–92.

Deyo, R. & D. L. Patrick 1989. Barriers to the use of health status measures in clinical investigation, patient care, and policy research. *Medical Care* **27**, Supplement, S254–S268.

Diener, E. 1984. Subjective well-being. *Psychological Bulletin* **95**, 542–75.

Doll H. A., N. Black, A. B. Flood, K. McPherson 1993. Criterion validation of the Nottingham Health Profile: patient views of surgery for benign prostatic hypertrophy. *Social Science and Medicine* **37**, 115–22.

Donaldson, C., A. Atkinson, J. Bond, K. Wright 1988. QALYs and long term care for people in the UK: scales for assessment of quality of life. *Age and Ageing* **17**, 379–86.

Donovan, J., S. Frankel, J. Eyles 1993. Assessing the need for health status measures. *Journal of Epidemiology and Community Health* **47**, 158–62.

Drewnowski, J. 1974. *On measuring and planning the quality of life*. The Hague: Mouton.

Dupuis, G. 1988. International perspectives on quality of life and cardiovascular disease: the quality of life systemic inventory. Paper presented at the workshop on quality of life in cardiovascular disease. Winston-Salem, NC.

Dupuy, H. J. 1978. Self representations of general psychological well-being of American adults. Paper presented at the American Public Health Association Meeting. Los Angeles, California.

Dworkin, R. 1981a. What is equality? Part I: Equality of welfare. *Philosophy and Public Affairs* **10**, 185–246.

Dworkin, R. 1981b. What is equality? Part II: Equality of resources. *Philosophy and Public Affairs* **10**, 283–345.

Edwards, A. 1957. *Techniques of attitude scale construction*. Englewood Cliffs, New

Jersey: Prentice Hall.

Elkinton, J. 1966. Medicine and the quality of life. *Annals of Internal Medicine* **64**, 711–14.

Ellwood, P. 1993. Rehabilitation, outcomes management, and health care reform. *Rehabilitation Management* **6**, 27–31.

Ellwood, P. 1988. Shattuck lecture-outcomes management: a technology of patient experience. *New England Journal of Medicine* **318**, 1549–56.

Elster, J. 1982. Sour grapes – Utilitarianism and the genesis of wants. In *Utilitarianism and beyond*, A. Sen & B. Williams (eds), 219–38. Cambridge: Cambridge University Press.

Enthoven, A. C. 1993. The history and principles of managed competition. *Health Affairs* **12**, 25–48.

Epstein, A. M., J. A. Hall, L. H. Son, L. Conant 1989. Using proxies to evaluate quality of life: can they provide information about patients' health status and satisfaction with medical care? *Medical Care* **27**, Supplement, 91–8.

Erickson, R. 1974. Welfare as a planning goal. *Acta Sociologica* **17**, 32–43.

Euroqol Group 1990. Euroqol – A new facility for the measurement of health-related quality of life. *Health Policy* **16**, 199–208.

Fadan, R. & A. Leplége 1992. Assessing quality of life: moral implications for clinical practice. *Medical Care* **30**, Supplement, 166–75.

Farquhar, M. 1991. Whose life is it anyway? The measurement of quality of life. Paper presented at The British Sociological Association Conference-Health and Society, University of Manchester.

Field, D. 1976. The social definition of illness. In *An Introduction to medical sociology*, D. Tuckett (ed.), 334–65. London: Tavistock.

Finlay, A. Y., G. K. Khan, D. K. Luscombe, M. S. Salek 1990. Validation of the Sickness Impact Profile and Psoriasis Disability Index in psoriasis. *British Journal of Dermatology* **123**, 751–6.

Fitzpatrick R., S. Newman, R. Lamb, M. Shipley 1988a. Social relationships and psychological well-being in rheumatoid arthritis. *Social Science and Medicine* **27** (4), 399–404.

Fitzpatrick R., S. Newman, R. Lamb, M. Shipley 1988b. A comparison of measures of health status in rheumatoid arthritis. *British Journal of Rheumatology* **28**, 201–6.

Fitzpatrick, R., J. Hinton, S. Newman, G. Scambler, J. Thompson (eds) 1984. *The experience of illness*. London: Tavistock Publications.

Fitzpatrick, R., S. Ziebland, C. Jenkinson. A. Mowat, A. Mowat 1993. A comparison of the sensitivity to change of several health status instruments in rheumatoid arthritis. *Journal of Rheumatology* **20**, 429–36.

Fitzpatrick, R., S. Ziebland, C. Jenkinson, A. Mowat, A. Mowat 1992. The importance of sensitivity to change as a criterion for selection of health status measures. *Quality in Health Care* **1**, 89–93.

Fitzpatrick, R., S. Ziebland, C. Jenkinson, A. Mowat, A. Mowat 1991. The social dimension of health status in rheumatoid arthritis. *International Disability Studies* **13**, 34–7.

Fletcher, A., P. McLoone, C. Bulpitt 1988. Quality of life on angina therapy: a randomized controlled trial of transdermal glyceryl trinitrate against placebo. *Lancet* **2**, 4–8.

Follick, M. J., T. W. Smith, D. K. Ahern 1985. The Sickness Impact Profile: global measure of disability in chronic low back pain. *Pain* **21**, 67–76.

Frankel, S., M. Williams, K. Nanchahal et al. 1991. *Total hip and knee joint replacement.* Bristol: University of Bristol (DHA project, Report 2).

Frankel, S. 1992. The epidemiology of indications. *Journal of Epidemiology and Community Health* **45**, 257–9.

Fries, J. F., P. W. Spitz, R. G. Kraines, H. R. Holman 1980. Measurement of patient outcome with arthritis. *Arthritis and Rheumatism* **23**, 137–45.

Fries, J. F., P. W. Spitz, D. Y. Young 1982. The dimensions of health outcomes: The Health Assessment Questionnaire, disability and pain scales. *Journal of Rheumatology* **9**, 789–93.

Froberg, D. & R. Kane 1989. Methodology for measuring health-state preferences-III Population and context effects. *Journal of Clinical Epidemiology* **42**, 585–92.

Gallagher, E. in press. Quality of life issues and the dialectic of medical progress illustrated by end-stage renal patients. *Advances in Medical Sociology.*

Garrett A. M., L. M. McDonald, D. A. Ruta, et al. 1993a. Towards measurement of outcome for patients with varicose veins. *Quality in Health Care* **2**, 5–10.

Garrett A. M., D. A. Ruta, M. I. Abdalla, et al. 1993b. The SF-36 health survey questionnaire: an outcome measure suitable for routine use within the NHS? *British Medical Journal* **306**, 1440–44.

Geigle, B. S. & S. B. Jones 1990. Outcomes measurement: a report from the front. *Inquiry* **27**, 7–13.

Gelijns, A. C. 1990. Comparing the development of drugs, devices, and clinical procedures. In *Modern methods of clinical investigation*, A. C. Gelijns (ed.), 147–201. Washington, DC: National Academy Press.

Gelijns, A. C. & S. O. Thier 1990. Medical technology development: an introduction to the innovation-evaluation nexus. In *Modern methods of clinical investigation*, A. C. Gelijns (ed.), 1–15. Washington, DC : National Academy Press.

Gilson, B. S., D. Erickson, C. T. Chavez, et al. 1980. A Chicano version of the Sickness Impact Profile. *Cultural and Medical Psychiatry* **4**, 137–50.

Glik, D. C. & J. J. Kronnenfeld 1989. Well rôles: sociological perspectives. In *Advances in the sociology of health care systems*. D. C. Wertz (ed.), 289–309. Greenwich, Connecticut: JAI Press.

Goldberg, D. P. 1972. *The detection of psychiatric illness by questionnaire.* London: Oxford University Press.

Goldsmith G. & M. Brodwick 1989. Assessing the functional status of older patients with chronic illness. *Family Medicine* **21**, 38–41.

Goldstein, M. & M. Hurwicz 1989. Psychological distress and perceived health status among elderly users of a health maintenance organization. *Journal of Gerontology* **44**, 154–6.

Gough, I. R., C. M. Furnival, L. Schilder, W. Grove 1983. Assessment of the quality of life of patients with advanced cancer. *European Journal of Clinical Oncology* **19**, 1161–5.

Granger, C., G. Albrecht, B. Hamilton 1979. Outcome of comprehensive medical rehabilitation: measurement by PULSES profile and the Barthel index. *Archives of Physical Medicine and Rehabilitation* **60**, 145–54.

Greenfield, S. & E. Nelson 1992. Recent developments and future issues in the use of health status assessment measures in clinical settings. *Medical Care* **30**, Supplement, MS23–MS41.

Greenwald, H. P. 1987. The specificity of quality of life measures among the seriously ill. *Medical Care* **25**, 642–51.

Grembowski, D., D. Patrick, P. Diehr, et al. 1993. Self-efficacy and health behavior among older adults. *Journal of Health and Social Behavior* **34**, 89–104.

Grimley Evans J. 1992. Quality of life assessments and elderly people. In *Measures of the Quality of Life*, A. Hopkins (ed.), 107–20. London: Royal College of Physicians of London.

Guyatt, G. H., L. B. Berman, M. Townsend, D. W. Taylor 1985. Should study subjects see their previous responses? *Journal of Chronic Diseases* **38**, 1003–7.

Guyatt, G. H., L. B. Berman, M. Townsend, S. O. Pugsley, L. W. Chambers 1987. A measure of quality of life for clinical trials in chronic lung disease. *Thorax* **42**, 773–8.

Guyatt, G., D. Feeny, D. Patrick 1993. Measuring health-related quality of life. *Annals of Internal Medicine* **118**, 622–9.

Guyatt, G., B. Kirschner, R. Jaeschke 1992. Measuring health status: what are the necessary measurement properties? *Journal of Clinical Epidemiology* **45**, 1341–5.

Guyatt, G., S. Van Zanten, D. Feeny, D. Patrick 1989. Measuring quality of life in clinical trials: a taxonomy and review. *Journal of the Canadian Medical Association* **140**, 1441–8.

Guyatt, G., S. Walter, G. Norman 1987. Measuring change over time: assessing the usefulness of evaluative instruments. *Journal of Chronic Diseases* **40**, 171–8.

Haga, H., T. Suzuki, S. Yasumura, H. Nagai, H. Amano, H. Shibata 1993. Factors predisposing to decline of physical function between ages 70 and 85 years. Paper presented at the XV International Congress of Gerontology, Budapest, Hungary.

Hart, G. L. & R. W. Evans 1987. The functional status of ESRD patients as measured by the Sickness Impact Profile. *Journal of Chronic Disease* **40**, Supplement 1, 117S–31S.

Harwood, R. H., P. Gompertz, P. Pound, S. Ebrahim (in press). Handicap one year after a stroke: validity of a new scale. *Journal of Neurology, Neurosurgery and Psychiatry*.

Hathaway, S. R. 1942. *The Minnesota multiphasic personality inventory*. Minneapolis: University of Minnesota Press.

Herzlich, C. 1973. *Health and illness*. London: Academic Press.

Herzlich, C. & J. Pierret 1987. *Illness and self in society*. Baltimore: The Johns Hopkins University Press.

Heyink, J. 1990. Adding years to your life or adding life to your years. *International Journal of Health Sciences* **1**, 45–50.

Hoeper, E. W., G. R. Nycz, L. Kessler, J. D. Burke, W. E. Pierce 1984. The usefulness of screening for mental illness. *Lancet* **1**, 33–5.

Hoinville, G. 1977. *The priority evaluator method*. Methodological working paper

3. Department of Social & Community Planning & Research, University of London.

Hunskaar S. & A. Vinsnes 1991. The quality of life in women with urinary incontinence as measured by the Sickness Impact Profile. *Journal of American Geriatric Society* **39**, 378–82.

Hunt, S. & J. McEwen 1980. The development of a subjective health indicator. *Sociology of Health and Illness* **2**, 231–46.

Hunt, S., J. McEwen, S. McKenna 1986. *Measuring health status*. London: Croom Helm.

Hunt, S. M., J. McEwen, S. P. McKenna 1985. Measuring health status: a new tool for clinicians and epidemiologists. *Journal of the Royal College of General Practitioners* **35**, 185–8.

Hunt, S. & S. McKenna 1991. *The Nottingham Health Profile user's manual, revised edition*. Manchester: Galen Research & Consultancy.

Hunt, S., S. McKenna, J. McEwen 1989. *The Nottingham Health Profile user's manual*. Manchester: Galen Research & Consultancy.

Hunt, S. M., S. P. McKenna, J. McEwen, et al. 1981. The Nottingham Health Profile: subjective health status and medical consultations. *Social Science and Medicine* **15**, 221–9.

Hunt, S. M., S. P. McKenna, J. McEwen, et al. 1980. A quantitative approach to perceived health status: a validation study. *Journal of Epidemiology and Community Health* **34**, 281–6.

Imershein, A., A. S. Hill, A. M. Reynolds. Workers' compensation system as a quality of life problem for workers' compensations claimants. *Advances in Medical Sociology*, in press.

Jacobsen, M. 1965. The use of rating scales in clinical research. *British Journal of Psychiatry* **111**, 545–6.

Janson-Bjerklie, S., S. Ferketich, P. Benner, G. Becker 1992. Clinical markers of asthma severity and risk: importance of subjective as well as objective factors. *Heart and Lung* **21**, 265–72.

Jenkinson, C. 1991. Why are we weighting? A critical examination of the use of item weights in a health status measure. *Social Science and Medicine* **32**, 1413–16.

Jenkinson, C., A. Coulter, L. Wright 1993a. Short form 36 (SF-36) health survey questionnaire: normative data for adults of working age. *British Medical Journal* **306**, 1437–40.

Jenkinson, C. & R. Fitzpatrick 1990. Measurement of health status in patients with chronic illness: Comparison of the Nottingham Health Profile and the General Health Questionnaire. *Family Practice* **7**, 121–4.

Jenkinson, C., R. Fitzpatrick, M. Argyle 1988. The Nottingham Health Profile: An analysis of its sensitivity in differentiating illness groups. *Social Science and Medicine* **27**, 1411–14.

Jenkinson, C., L. Wright, A. Coulter 1994. Criterion validity and reliability of the SF-36 in a population sample. *Quality of Life Research* **3**, 7–12.

Jenkinson, C., L. Wright, A. Coulter 1993b. *Quality of life measurement in health care: a review of measures, and population norms for the UK SF-36*. Oxford: Health Services Research Unit.

Jenkinson, C., S. Ziebland, R. Fitzpatrick, A. Mowat, A. Mowat 1991. Sensitivity to change of weighted and unweighted versions of two Health Status Measures. *International Journal of Health Sciences* **2**, 189–94.

Jenkinson, C., S. Ziebland, R. Fitzpatrick, A. Mowat, A. Mowat 1993c. Hospitalisation and its influence upon results from Health Status Questionnaires. *International Journal of Health Sciences* **4**, 13–19.

Jette, A. M. 1980. Health status indicators: their utility in chronic-disease evaluation. *Journal of Chronic Disease* **33**, 567–79.

Jette, A. M., A. R. Cleary, P. D. Calteins, et al. 1986. The Functional Status Questionnaire: reliability and validity when used in primary care. *Journal of General and Internal Medicine* **1**, 143–9.

Johnson, R. J. & F. D. Wolinsky 1993. The structure of health status among older adults: disease, disability, functional limitation, and perceived health. *The Journal of Health and Social Behavior* **34**, 105–21.

Johnstone, A. & D. P. Goldberg 1976. Psychiatric screening in general practice. *Lancet* **1**, 605–8.

Jones, P. W. 1991. Quality of life measurement for patients with diseases of the airways. *Thorax* **46** (9), 676–82.

Jones, P. W. 1988. Measuring the quality of life of patients with respiratory disease. In *Quality of life: assessment and application*, S. R. Walker & R. M. Rosser (eds), 235–51. Lancaster: MTP Press.

Jones, P. W., C. M. Baveystock, P. Littlejohns 1989. Relationship between general health measured with the Sickness Impact Profile and respiratory symptoms, physiological measures, and mood in patients with chronic airflow limitation. *American Review of Respiratory Disease* **140**, 1538–3.

Kahneman, D. & C. Varey 1991. Notes on the psychology of utility. In *Interpersonal comparisons of well-being*, J. Elster & J. Roemer (eds), 127–63. Cambridge: Cambridge University Press.

Kane, R. L. 1987. Commentary: Functional Assessment Questionnaire for geriatric patients – or the clinical Swiss army knife. *Medical Care*, Supplement, S95–S99.

Kaplan, R., J. Bush, C. Berry 1976. Health status: types of validity and the index of well-being. *Health Services Research* **11**, 478–507.

Kaplan, R. M. & J. P. Anderson 1988. The Quality of Well-Being Scale: rationale for a single quality of life index. In *Quality of life: assessment and application*, S. R. Walker & R. M. Rosser (eds), 51–77. Lancaster: MTP Press.

Katz, J. N., M. G. Larson, C. Phillips, A. Fossel, M. H. Liang 1992. Comparative measurement sensitivity of short and longer health status instruments. *Medical Care* **30**, 917–25.

Katz, S. 1987. The science of quality of life. *Journal of Chronic Diseases* **40**, 459–63.

Katz, S. & C. A. Akpom 1976. Index of ADL. *Medical Care* **14**, 116–18.

Katz, S., A. Ford, B. Moskowitz, B. Jackson, M. Jaffee 1963. Studies of illness in the aged: the index of ADL: a standardized measure of biological and psychological function. *Journal of the American Medical Association* **185**, 914–19.

Kazis, L. E., J. J. Anderson, R. F. Meenan 1990. Health status as a predictor of mortality in rheumatoid arthritis: a five-year study. *Journal of Rheumatology* **17**,

609–13.

Kazis L. E., J. J. Anderson, R. F. Meenan 1989. Effect sizes for interpreting changes in health status. *Medical Care* 27, Supplement, 178–89.

Keith R. A., C. V. Granger, B. B. Hamilton, F. S. Sherwin 1987. The Functional Independence Measure: A new tool for rehabilitation. *Advances in Clinical Rehabilitation* 1, 6–18.

Kelly, T. L. 1927. *Interpretation of educational measurements*. Yonkers: World Book Publishing.

Kerlinger, F. N. 1973. *Foundations of behavioral research*. New York: Holt, Rinehart & Winston.

Kind, P. 1982. A comparison of two models for scaling health indicators. *International Journal of Epidemiology* 11, 271–5.

Kind P. & R. Carr-Hill 1987. The Nottingham Health Profile: a useful tool for epidemiologists? *Social Science & Medicine* 25, 905–10.

Kraus, N. 1990. *The InterStudy Quality Edge 1 (1)*. Excelsior, MN: InterStudy.

Krenz, C., E. B. Larson, D. M. Buchner, C. G. Canfield 1988. Characterising patients' dysfunction in Alzheimers-type dementia. *Medical Care* 29, 453–61.

Lane D. 1988. Disabling breathlessness. In *Disabling diseases*, A. O. Frank & G. P. McGuire (eds), 79–97. London: Heinemann.

Larson, J. 1993. The measurement of social well-being. *Social Indicators Research* 28, 285–96.

Laughlin, J., C. Granger, B. Hamilton 1992. Outcomes measurement for medical rehabilitation. *Rehabilitation Management* 5, 57–8.

Levine, S. 1987. The changing terrains in medical sociology: emergent concern with quality of life. *Journal of Health and Social Behavior* 28, 1–6.

Liang, M. H., K. E. Cullen, M. G. Larson, et al. 1986. Cost effectiveness of total joint arthroplasty. *Arthritis and Rheumatism* 29, 937–43.

Liang, M. H., K. Cullen, M. Larson 1982. In search of a more perfect mousetrap (Health status or quality of life instrument). *Journal of Rheumatology* 9, 775–9.

Liang, M., A. Fossel, M. Larson 1990. Comparisons of five health status instruments for orthopaedic evaluation. *Medical Care* 28, 632–42.

Liang, M. H., M. G. Larson, K. E. Cullen, J. A. Schwartz 1985. Comparative measurement efficiency and sensitivity of five health status instruments for arthritis research. *Arthritis and Rheumatism* 28, 542–7.

Lydick, E. & R. S. Epstein 1993. Interpretation of quality of life changes. *Quality of Life Research* 2, 221–6.

MacIntyre, S. 1986a. The patterning of health by social position in contemporary Britain: Directions for sociological research. *Social Science and Medicine* 23, 393–415.

MacIntyre, S. 1986b. Health and illness. In *Key variables in social investigation*, R.G. Burgess (ed.), 99-122. London: Routledge & Kegan Paul.

Magaziner, J., E. M. Simonsick, T. M. Kashner, J. R. Hebel 1988. Patient-proxy response comparability on measures of patient health and functional status. *Journal of Clinical Epidemiology* 41, 1065–74.

Mahoney, F. & D. Barthel 1965. Functional evaluation: the Barthel index. *Maryland State Medical Journal* 14, 61–5.

REFERENCES

Mant, D. & G. Fowler 1990. Mass screening: theory and ethics. *British Medical Journal* **300**, 916–18.

Marks, D. F. & B. G. Chipperfield 1992. A health and lifestyle survey of Londoners: preliminary data from the Bloomsbury and Islington health and lifestyle survey. Symposium on Health Behaviour VIth European Health Psychology Society Conference, Leipzig, Germany.

Markson, L. E., D. B. Nash, D. Z. Louis, J. S. Gonnella 1991. Clinical outcomes management and disease staging. *Evaluation and the Health Professions* **14**, 201–27.

Marshall, V. W. 1993. Social models of aging. Paper presented at the XVth International Congress of Gerontology, Budapest, Hungary.

McDowell, I. & C. Newell 1987. *Measuring health: a guide to rating scales and questionnaires.* New York: Oxford University Press.

McFarlane, A. H., K. A. Neale, G. R. Norman, R. G. Roy, D. L. Streiner 1981. Methodological issues in developing a scale to measure social support. *Schizophrenia Bulletin* **7**, 90–99.

McGee, H. M., C. A. O'Boyle, A. Hickey, K. O'Malley, C. R. B. Joyce 1991. Assessing the quality of life of the individual: the SEIQoL with a healthy and a gastroenterology unit population. *Psychological Medicine* **21**, 749–59.

McHorney C. A., J. E. Ware, J. F. R. Lu, in press. The MOS 36-item short-form health survey (SF-36): III. Tests of data quality, scaling assumptions and reliability across diverse patient groups. *Medical Care.*

McHorney, C. A., J. E. Ware, J. F. R. Lu (1993) The MOS 36-item short-form health survey (SF-36): II. Psychometric and clinical tests of validity in measuring physical and mental health constructs. *Medical Care* **31**, 247–63.

McHorney, C. A., J. E. Ware, W. Rogers, A. E. Raczek, J. F. R. Lu 1992. The validity and relative precision of MOS short and long form health status measures and Dartmouth COOP charts: results from the Medical Outcomes Study. *Medical Care* **5**, Supplement, MS253–MS265.

McIver, J. P. & E. G. Carmines 1981. *Unidimensional scaling.* Sage University Paper series: Quantitative Applications in the Social Sciences. London: Sage.

McKenna, S. P., S. M. Hunt, J. McEwen 1981. Weighting the seriousness of perceived health problems using Thurstone's method of paired comparisons. *International Journal of Epidemiology* **10**, 93–7.

McKenna, S., S. Hunt, A. Tennant. 1993 The development of a patient-completed index of distress from the Nottingham Health Profile: A new measure for use in cost-utility studies. *Journal of Medical Economics* **6**, 13–24.

McKenna, S. & R. L. Payne 1989. Comparison of the General Health Questionnaire and the Nottingham Health Profile in a study of unemployed and re-employed men. *Family Practice* **6**, 3–8.

McSweeny, A. J., R. K. Heaton, I. Grant, et al. 1980. Chronic obstructive pulmonary disease: socioemotional adjustment and life quality. *Chest* **77**, Supplement, 309–11.

McSweeny, A. J., I. Grant, R. K. Heaton, K. M. Adams, R. M. Timms 1982. Life Quality of patients with chronic obstructive pulmonary disease. *Archives of Internal Medicine* **144**, 473–8.

McSweeny, A. J. & K. T. Labuhn 1990. Chronic obstructive pulmonary disease. In *Quality of life assessments in clinical trials*, B. Spilker (ed.), 391–417. New York: Raven Press.

Meenan, R. F. 1982. The AIMS approach to health status measurement: conceptual background and measurement properties. *Journal of Rheumatology* **9**, 785–8.

Meenan, R. F., J. J. Anderson, L. E. Kazis, et al. 1984. Outcome assessment in clinical trials: evidence for the sensitivity of a health status measure. *Arthritis and Rheumatism* **27**, 1344–52.

Meenan, R. F., P. M. Gertman, J. H. Mason 1980. Measuring health status in arthritis: the arthritis impact measurement scales. *Arthritis & Rheumatism* **23**, 146–52.

Meenan, R. F., P. M. Gertman, J. H. Mason, et al. 1982. The arthritis impact measurement scales: further investigations of a health status measure. *Arthritis and Rheumatism* **25**, 1048–53.

Meenan, R. F., J. H. Mason, J. J. Anderson, et al. 1992. AIMS2: The content and properties of a revised and expanded arthritis impact measurement scales health status questionnaire. *Arthritis and Rheumatism* **35**, 1–10.

Melzack, R. 1973. *The puzzle of pain*. New York: Basic Books.

Mohr, L. B. 1992. *Impact analysis for program evaluation*. Newbury Park, California: Sage.

Muller, C. F. 1990. *Health and gender*. New York: Russell Sage Foundation.

Najman, J. & S. Levine 1981. Evaluating the impact of medical care and technologies on the quality of life: a review and critique. *Social Science and Medicine* **15**, 107–16.

Nelson, E., J. Landgraf, R. Hays, J. Wasson, J. Kirk 1990. The functional status of patients: how can it be measured in physicians' offices? *Medical Care* **28**, 1111–1126.

Neugarten, B. L., R. J. Havighurst, S. S. Tobin 1961. The measurement of life satisfaction. *Journal of Gerontology* **16**, 134–43.

Norton, P. A., L. D. MacDonald, P. M. Sedgwick, S. L. Stanton 1988. Distress and delay associated with urinary incontinence, frequency, and urgency in women. *British Medical Journal* **297**, 1187–9.

Nunnally, J. C. 1978. *Psychometric theory*, second edition. New York: McGraw Hill.

O'Boyle, C. A., H. McGee, A. Hickey, C. R. B. Joyce, K. O'Malley 1993. *The schedule for the evaluation of individual quality of life (SEIQoL): Administration manual.* Dublin: Department of Psychology, Medical School, Royal College of Surgeons in Ireland.

O'Boyle, C. A., H. McGee, A. Hickey, K. O'Malley, C. R. B. Joyce 1992. Individual quality of life in patients undergoing hip replacement. *Lancet* **339**, 1088–91.

O'Brien B. J. 1988. Assessment of treatment in heart disease. In *Measuring health: a practical approach*, G. Teeling-Smith (ed.), 191–211. Chichester: John Wiley.

O'Brien, B. J., N. R. Banner, S. Gibson, M. H. Yacoub 1988. The Nottingham Health Profile as a measure of quality of life following combined heart and lung transplantation. *Journal of Epidemiology and Community Health* **42**, 232–4.

Ott, C. R., E. S. Sivarajan, K. Newton, et al. 1983. A controlled randomized study of early cardiac rehabilitation: the Sickness Impact Profile as an assessment tool. *Heart Lung* **12**, 162–70.

Oxford English Dictionary 1982. *Supplement*. Oxford: Clarendon Press.

Patrick, D. L. & P. E. Erickson 1993. *Health status and health policy: allocating resources to health care*. Oxford: Oxford University Press.

Patrick, D. & H. Peach (eds) 1989. *Disablement in the community*. Oxford: Oxford University Press.

Patrick, D. L., H. Peach, I. Gregg 1982. Disablement and care: a comparison of patient views and general practitioner knowledge. *Journal of the Royal College of General Practitioners* **32**, 429–34.

Patrick, D. L., Y. Sittampalam, S. Sommerville, S. Carter, M. Bergner 1985. A cross-cultural comparison of health status values. *American Journal of Public Health* **71** (2), 1402–7.

Pearse, I. H. & L. H. Crocker 1943. *The Peckham Experiment: a study of the living structure of society*. London: Allen & Unwin.

Pigou, A. C. 1920. *The economics of welfare*. London: Macmillan.

Pill, R. & N. C. H. Stott 1982. Concept of illness causation and responsibility: some preliminary data from a sample of working class mothers. *Social Science and Medicine* **16**, 43–52.

Pincus, T., L. Callahan, R. Brooks, et al. 1989. Self-report questionnaire scores in rheumatoid arthritis compared with traditional physical radiographic and laboratory measures. *Annals of Internal Medicine* **150**, 59–62.

Pincus, T., J. A. Summey, S. Soraci Jr, K. Wallston, N. P. Hummon 1983. Assessment of patient satisfaction in activities of daily living using a modified Stanford Health Assessment Questionnaire. *Arthritis and Rheumatism* **26**, 1346–53.

Policy PC. 1986. Software for judgement analysis: version 2.0. Reference manual, 1st edn, available from Executive Decision Services, PO Box 9102, Albany, New York.

Pollard, W. E., R. A. Bobbitt, M. Bergner, D. P. Martin, B. S. Gilson 1976. The Sickness Impact Profile: reliability of a health status measure. *Medical Care* **14**, 146–55.

Pope, A. & A. Tarlov (eds) 1991. *Disability in America: toward a national agenda for prevention*. Washington, DC: National Academy Press.

Potts, S. 1992. The QALY and why it should be resisted. In *Philosophy and health care*, E. Mathews & M. Menlowe (eds), 43–63. Aldershot: Avebury.

Presant, C. A. 1984. Quality of life in cancer patients. Who measures what? *American Journal of Clinical Oncology* **7**, 571–3.

Prigatano, G. P., E. C. Wright, D. Levin 1984. Quality of life and its predictors in patients with mild hypoxaemia and chronic obstructive pulmonary disease. *Archives of Internal Medicine* **144**, 1613–19.

Procidano, M. E. & K. Heller 1983. Measures of perceived social support from friends and from family: three validation studies. *American Journal of Community Psychology* **11**, 1–24.

Quebec Task Force 1987. Scientific approach to the assessment and management of activity-related spinal disorders. A monograph for clinicians. Report of the Quebec Task Force on spinal disorders. *Spine*, Supplement, **12**, 1–59.

Quirk, F. & P. Jones 1990. Perception of distress due to symptoms and effects of asthma on daily living and an investigation of possible influential factors. *Clinical Science* **79**, 17–21.

Radloff, L. 1977. The CES-D scale. *Applied Psychological Measurement* **1**, 385–401.

Rawls, J. 1982. Social unity and primary goods. In *Utilitarianism and beyond,* A. Sen & B. Williams (eds), 159–85. Cambridge: Cambridge University Press.

Read, J. L., R. J. Quinn, M. A. Hoefer 1987. Measuring overall health: an evaluation of three important approaches. *Journal of Chronic Disease* **40**, Supplement, 7–21.

Reisine, S. T., J. Fertig, J. Weber, S. Leder 1989. Impact of dental conditions on patient's quality of life. *Community Dentistry and Oral Epidemiology* **17**, 7–10.

Reuben, D. B., L. V. Rubenstein, S. H. Hirsch, R. Hays 1992. The value of functional status as a predictor of mortality: results of a prospective study. *American Journal of Medicine* **93**, 663–9.

Richardson, J. 1992. Cost-utility analyses in health care: present status and future issues. In *Researching health care,* J. Daly, I. McDonald, E. Willis (eds), 21–44. London: Routledge.

Riessman, C. K. 1983. Women and medicalization: a new perspective. *Social Policy* **14**, 3–18.

Robinson, I. 1990. Personal narratives, social careers and medical courses: analyzing life trajectories in autobiographies of people with multiple sclerosis. *Social Science and Medicine* **30**, 1173–86.

Rolland M. & R. Morris 1983. A study of the natural history of back pain: part I: development of a reliable and sensitive measure of disability in low-back pain. *Spine* **8**, 141–4.

Rosser, R., M. Cottee, R. Rabin, C. Selai 1992. Index of health-related quality of life. In *Measures of the Quality of Life,* A. Hopkins (ed.), 81–90. London: Royal College of Physicians of London.

Rosser, R. M., J. Denford, A. Heslop, et al. 1983. Breathlessness and psychiatric morbidity in chronic bronchitis and emphysema: a study of psychotherapeutic management. *Psychological Medicine* **13**, 93–110.

Rosser, R. & P. Kind 1978. A scale of valuations of states of illness – is there a social consensus? *International Journal of Epidemiology* **1**, 361–8.

Rossi, P. H. & H. E. Freeman 1989. *Evaluation: a systematic approach.* Newbury Park: Sage.

Rothman, M. L., S. C. Hedrick, K. A. Bulcrot, D. H. Hickman, L. Z. Rubenstein 1991. The validity of proxy-generated scores as measures of patient health status. *Medical Care* **29**, 115–24.

Rowan, K. 1992. *Outcome comparisons of intensive care units in Great Britain and Ireland using the APACHE II method.* DPhil thesis, University of Oxford.

Rubenstein, L. V., D. R. Calkins, R. T. Young, et al. 1989. Improving patient function: a randomized trial of functional disability screening. *Annals of Internal Medicine* **111**, 836–42.

Ruta, D. A., A. M. Garratt, M. Leng, I. T. Russell, L. M. Macdonald, in press, a. A new approach to the measurement of quality of life: the patient generated index (PGI). *Medical Care.*

Ruta D., A. Garratt, M. Abdalla, K. Buckingham, I. Russell 1993. The SF-36 health survey questionnaire: a valid measure of health status. *British Medical Journal* **307**, 448.

Ruta, D. A., A. M. Garratt, D. Wardlaw, I. T. Russell, in press, b. Developing a valid and reliable measure of health outcome for patients with low back pain. *Spine*.

Sackett, D. L., L. W. Chambers, A. S. McPherson, C. H. Goldsmith, R. G. McAuley 1977. The development and application of indices of health: general methods and a summary of results. *American Journal of Public Health* **67**, 423–8.

Scanlon, T. 1991. The moral basis of interpersonal comparison. In *Interpersonal comparisons of well-being*, J. Elster & J. Roemer (eds), 17–44. Cambridge: Cambridge University Press.

Scanlon, T. 1993. Value, desire, and quality of life. In *The quality of life*, M. Nussbaum & A. Sen (eds), 185–200. Oxford: Clarendon Press.

Schumacher, M., M. Olschewski, G. Schulgen 1991. Assessment of quality of life in clinical trials. *Statistics in Medicine* **10**, 1915–30.

Sen, A. 1993. Positional objectivity. *Philosophy and Public Affairs* **22**, 126–45.

Sen, A. 1992. *Inequality re-examined*. Oxford: Clarendon.

Sen, A. 1990. Justice: Means versus freedom. *Philosophy and Public Affairs* **19**, 111–21.

Sen, A. 1982. *Equality of what? Choice, welfare and measurement*. Oxford: Blackwell.

Sen, A. & B. Williams 1982. *Utilitarianism and beyond*. Cambridge: Cambridge University Press.

Sheldon, T. 1993. Reliability of the SF-36 remains uncertain. *British Medical Journal* **307**, 125–6.

Sherbourne, C. D. 1992a. Social functioning: social activity limitations measure. See Stewart & Ware (1992), 173–81.

Sherbourne, C. D. 1992b. Pain measures. See Stewart & Ware (1992), 220–34.

Sherbourne, C. D., A. L. Stewart, K. B. Wells 1992. Rôle functioning measures. See Stewart & Ware (1992), 205–19.

Slevin, M., H. Plant, D. Lynch, et al. 1988. Who should measure quality of life, the doctor or the patient? *British Journal of Cancer* **57**, 109–12.

Spilker, B. 1990. *Quality of life assessment in clinical trials*. New York: Raven Press.

Spitzer, W. O. 1987. Keynote address: state of science 1986: quality of life and functional status as target variables for research. *Journal of Chronic Diseases* **40**, 465–74.

Spitzer, W. O., A. J. Dobson, J. Hall, et al. 1981. Measuring the quality of life of cancer patients: a concise QL-Index for use by physicians. *Journal of Chronic Diseases* **34**, 585–97.

Sprangers, M. A. & N. K. Aaronson 1992. The rôle of health care providers and significant others in evaluating the quality of life of patients with chronic disease: a review. *Journal of Clinical Epidemiology* **45**, 743–60.

Stanton, A. L. 1987. Determinants of adherence to medical regimens by hypertensive patients. *Journal of Behavioral Medicine* **10**, 377–94.

Starr, P. 1992. *The logic of health-care reform*. Knoxville, Tennessee: Whittle Direct Books.

Stevens, S. 1951. Mathematics, measurement and psychophysics. In *Handbook of experimental psychology*, S. Stevens (ed.), 1–14. New York: Wiley.

Stewart, A. L., S. Greenfield, R. D. Hays, et al. 1989. Functional status and well-being of patients with chronic conditions: results from the Medical Outcomes Study. *Journal of the American Medical Association* **262**, 907–13.

Stewart, A. L., R. D. Hays, J. E. Ware 1992a. Methods of constructing health measures. See Stewart & Ware (1992), 67–85.

Stewart, A. L., R. D. Hays, J. E. Ware 1992b. Methods of validating health measures. See Stewart & Ware (1992), 309–24.

Stewart, A. L., R. D. Hays, J. E. Ware 1992c. Health perceptions, energy/fatigue, and health distress measures. See Stewart & Ware (1992), 143–72.

Stewart, A. L., R. D. Hays, J. E. Ware 1988. The MOS short form general health survey. *Medical Care* 26, 724–35.

Stewart, A. L. & C. J. Kamberg 1992. Physical functioning measures. See Stewart & Ware (1992), 86–101.

Stewart, A. L., C. D. Sherbourne, R. D. Hays, et al. 1992d. Summary and discussion of MOS measures. See Stewart & Ware (1992), 345–72.

Stewart, A. L., J. E. Ware, R. H. Brook 1978. *Conceptualization and measurement of health for adults in the health insurance study: Volume 2*. Santa Monica, California: RAND Corporation.

Stewart A. L. & J. E. Ware 1992. *Measuring functioning and well-being: the medical outcomes approach*. London: Duke University Press.

Stewart, A. L., J. E. Ware, C. D. Sherbourne, K. B. Wells 1992e. Psychological distress/well-being and cognitive functioning measures. See Stewart & Ware (1992), 102–42.

Stewart, T. R. 1988. Judgement analysis: procedures. In *Human judgement: the social judgement theory view*, B. Brehmer & C. R. B. Joyce (eds), 41–75. Amsterdam: North-Holland.

Stokes, J. P. 1983. Predicting satisfaction with social support from social network structure. *American Journal of Community Psychology* **11**, 141–52.

Stoller, E. 1984. Self-assessments of health by the elderly: the impact of informal assistance. *Journal of Health and Social Behavior* **25**: 260–70.

Streiner, D. L. & G. R. Norman 1989. *Health Measurement scales: a practical guide to their development and use*. Oxford: Oxford University Press.

Sullivan, F. M., R. C. Eagers, K. Lynch, J. H. Barber 1987. Assessment of disability caused by rheumatic diseases in general practice. *Annals of the Rheumatic Diseases* **46**, 598–600.

Tarlov, A. R. 1983. Shattuck lecture – the increasing supply of physicians, the changing structure of the health services system, and the future practice of medicine. *New England Journal of Medicine* **308**, 1235–44.

Tarlov A. R., J. E. Ware, S. Greenfield, et al. 1989. The Medical Outcomes Study: an application of methods for monitoring the results of medical care. *Journal of the American Medical Association* **262**, 925–30.

Teeling-Smith, G. 1988. *Measuring health: a practical approach*. Chichester: John Wiley.

Temkin, N. R., S. Dikmen, J. Machamer, A. McLean 1989. General versus disease specific measures: further work on the Sickness Impact Profile for head injury.

Medical Care **27**, Supplement, 544–53.

Temkin, N. R., A. McLean, S. Dikmen, et al. 1988. Development and evaluation of modifications to the Sickness Impact Profile for head injury. *Journal of Clinical Epidemiology* **41**, 47–57.

Thunhurst, C. & A. MacFarlane 1992. Monitoring the health of urban populations: what statistics do we need? *Journal of the Royal Statistical Society*, Series A **155**, 1–21.

Thurstone, L. 1928. Attitudes can be measured. *American Journal of Sociology* **33**, 529–54.

Thurstone, L. 1927. A law of comparative judgement. *Psychological Review* **34**, 273–86.

Thurstone, L. & E. J. Chave 1929. *The measurement of attitude*. Chicago: University of Chicago Press.

Tuckett, D., M. Boulton, C. Olson, A. Williams 1985. *Meetings between experts*. London: Tavistock.

Tugwell, C., C. Bombardier, W. Buchanan, et al. 1990. Methotrexate in rheumatoid arthritis: impact on quality of life assessed by traditional standard item and individualized patient preference health status questionnaires. *Archives of Internal Medicine* **150**, 59–62.

Tugwell, C., C. Bombardier, W. Buchanan, et al. 1987. The MACTAR patient preference disability questionnaire. An individualised functional priority approach for assessing improvement in physical disability in clinical trials in rheumatoid arthritis. *Journal of Rheumatology* **14**, 446–51.

Vandenburg, M. J. 1988. Measuring the quality of life of patients with angina. In *Quality of life: assessment and application*, S. R. Walker & R. M. Rosser (eds), 267–77. Lancaster: MTP Press.

Villar, J., U. Farnot, F. Barros 1992. A randomized trial of psychosocial support during high-risk pregnancies. *New England Journal of Medicine* **327**, 1266–71.

Waitzkin, H. 1991. *The politics of medical encounters*. New Haven, Connecticut: Yale University Press.

Walker, S. R. & R. M. Rosser (eds) *Quality of life: assessment and application*. Lancaster: MTP Press

Ware, J. E. 1993. Measuring patients' views: the optimum outcome measure. SF-36: a valid, reliable assessment of health from the patient's point of view. *British Medical Journal* **306**, 1429–30.

Ware, J. E. 1992. Measures for a new era of health assessment. See Stewart & Ware (1992), 3-11.

Ware J. E. 1987. Standards for validating health measures: definition and content. *Journal of Chronic Diseases* **40**, 473–80.

Ware, J. E., R. H. Brook, A. Davies-Avery 1980. *Conceptualization and measurement of health for adults in the health insurance study: Volume I Model of health and methodology*. Santa Monica: RAND Corporation.

Ware, J. E., R. H. Brook, A. R. Davies, K. N. Lohr 1981. Choosing measures of health status for individuals in general populations. *American Journal of Public Health* **71**, 620–25.

Ware, J. E., R. Brook, W. Rogers, et al. 1986. Comparison of health outcomes at a health maintenance organisation with those of fee-for-service care. *Lancet* **1**, 1017–22.

Ware J. E., E. C. Nelson, C. D. Sherbourne, A. L. Stewart 1992a. Preliminary tests of a 6-item general health survey: a patient application. See Stewart & Ware (1992), 291–308.

Ware, J. E. & C. D. Sherbourne 1992. The MOS 36-Item Short-Form Health Survey (SF-36). I: Conceptual framework and item selection. *Medical Care* **30** (6), 473–83.

Ware J. E., C. D. Sherbourne, A. R. Davies 1992b. Developing and testing the MOS 20-item short-form health survey: a general population survey. See Stewart & Ware (1992), 277–90.

Ware J. E., K. K. Snow, M. Kosinski, B. Gandek 1993. *SF-36 Health Survey: manual and interpretation guide*. Boston: The Health Institute, New England Medical Center.

Wasson, J., A. Keller, L., Rubenstein, et al. 1992. Benefits and obstacles of health status assessment in ambulatory settings: the clinician's point of view. *Medical Care*, **30** Supplement, MS42–MS49.

Watt-Watson, J. H. & J. E. Graydon 1989. Sickness Impact Profile: a measure of dysfunction with chronic pain patients. *Journal of Pain Symptoms and Management* **4**, 152–6.

Wechsler, D. 1945. A standardized memory scale for clinical use. *Journal of Psychology* **19**, 87–95.

Weiner, E. A. & B. J. Stewart 1984. *Assessing individuals*. Boston: Little Brown.

Wells K. B., A. L. Stewart, R. D. Hays, et al. 1989. The functioning and well-being of depressed patients: results from the Medical Outcomes Study. *Journal of the American Medical Association* **262**, 914–19.

Wenger, N. K., M. E. Mattson, C. D. Furberg et al. (eds), 1984. *Assessment of quality of life in clinical trials of cardiovascular therapies*. New York: Le Jacq Publishing.

Wennberg, J. E. 1990a. Outcomes research, cost containment, and the fear of health care rationing. *The New England Journal of Medicine* **323**, 1202–5.

Wennberg, J. E. 1990b. What is outcomes research? In A. C. Gelijns (ed.), *Modern methods of clinical investigation*. Washington, DC: National Academy Press.

Wilkin, D., L. Hallam, M. Doggett 1992. *Measures of need and outcome for primary health care*. Oxford: Oxford University Press.

Wilkin, D., L. Hallam, M. Doggett 1993. *Measures of need and outcome for primary health care*, revd edn. Oxford: Oxford University Press.

Williams, A. 1992. Review of A. L. Stewart and J. E. Ware (eds), Measuring functioning and well-being: the Medical Outcomes Study approach. *Health Economics* **1**, 4.

Williams, A. 1985. Economics of coronary artery bypass grafting. *British Medical Journal* **291**, 326–9.

Williams, A. & P. Kind 1992. The present state of play about QALYs. In *Measures of the quality of life*, A. Hopkins (ed.), 21–34. London: Royal College of Physicians of London.

Williams S. J. 1993. *Chronic respiratory illness*. London: Routledge.

Williams S. J. 1990. *The consequences of chronic respiratory illness: a sociological study*.

Doctoral dissertation: University of London.

Williams S. J. & M. R. Bury 1989a. Impairment, disability and handicap in chronic respiratory illness. *Social Science and Medicine* **29**, 609–17.

Williams S. J. & M. R. Bury 1989b. Breathtaking: the consequences of chronic respiratory disorder. *International Disability Studies* **11**, 114–20.

Wilson, J. D., E. Braunwold, K. J. Isselbacher, et al. 1991. *Harrison's principles of internal medicine*, 12th edn. New York: McGraw-Hill.

Wilson, T. C. 1993. Urbanism and kinship bonds: a test of four generalizations. *Social Forces* **71**, 703–12.

Wolfe, F. & T. Pincus 1991. Standard self-report questionnaires in routine clinical and research practice – an opportunity for patients and rheumatologists. *Journal of Rheumatology* **18**, 643-4.

World Health Organisation 1984. *Uses of epidemiology in aging: report of a scientific group*. Technical Report Series 706. Geneva: WHO.

World Health Organisation 1958. *The First Ten Years of the World Health Organisation*. Geneva: WHO.

World Health Organisation 1947. The constitution of the world health organization. *WHO Chronicle* 1, 13.

World Health Organisation 1948. *WHO Constitution*. Geneva: WHO.

Wright, L, D. Harwood, A. Coulter 1992. Health and lifestyles in the Oxford region. Oxford: Health Services Research Unit.

Young, J. B. & M. A. Chamberlain 1987. The contribution of the Stanford Health Assessment Questionnaire in rheumatology clinics. *Clinical Rehabilitation* **1**, 97–100.

Ziebland, S., R. Fitzpatrick, C. Jenkinson 1993. Tacit models of disability in Health Assessment Questionnaires. *Social Science and Medicine* **37**, 69–75.

Ziebland, S., R. Fitzpatrick, C. Jenkinson 1992a. Assessing short term outcome. *Quality in Health Care* **1**, 141–2.

Ziebland, S., R. Fitzpatrick, C. Jenkinson, A. Mowat, A. Mowat 1992b. Comparison of two approaches to measuring change in health status in rheumatoid arthritis: The Health Assessment Questionnaire (HAQ) and the Modified HAQ. *Annals of the Rheumatic Diseases* **51**, 1202–5.

Zung, W. W. K. 1983. A self rating pain and distress scale. *Psychosomatics* **24**, 887–94.

Index